The C.
Diet

D0282170

If you're on a diet that c   drates, this book is designed to help you maintain the discipline you'll need to succeed with your diet.

Take your Diary with you everywhere and record everything you eat and drink. Using the compact carbohydrate gram counter (pages 135–174), compute the carbs for each item and total them up for the day. If you write down everything as you eat it, the very act of recording it will make you think twice about what and when you are eating. In addition, by reviewing the page, you can see where the "danger spots" in the day are and make the diet corrections accordingly, using the daily comments page.

Before going on any diet, consult with your doctor. Then determine your desired weight and how many carbohydrate grams a day you want to limit yourself to. While the purpose of this book is not to advocate any specific low-carbohydrate diet, there are some overall guidelines to use. When you begin your diet, your daily carbohydrate intake should be very low. When you reach certain goals, you may wish to increase your carbs to what most diets refer to as the "maintenance level," still a comparatively low count, but less rigid than the initial weeks.

Start by recording your goals on page 6 and chart your diet every seven days in the Weekly Progress Report. Note your weight and measurement changes and your plans for the coming week. You'll also find space to record your exercise program. If you're not already exercising on a regular basis, start now. Exercising helps tone and tighten your body as it reaches new proportions.

Good luck and good dieting.

C.T.N.

Books by Corinne T. Netzer

THE CORINNE T. NETZER BRAND-NAME
CALORIE COUNTER

THE COMPLETE BOOK OF FOOD COUNTS

THE CORINNE T. NETZER CHOLESTEROL COUNTER

THE CORINNE T. NETZER CARBOHYDRATE
COUNTER

THE CORINNE T. NETZER CARBOHYDRATE
AND FIBER COUNTER

THE CORINNE T. NETZER CARBOHYDRATE
DIETER'S DIARY

THE CORINNE T. NETZER DIETER'S DIARY

THE CORINNE T. NETZER ENCYCLOPEDIA
OF FOOD VALUES

THE CORINNE T. NETZER FAT COUNTER

THE CORINNE T. NETZER FIBER COUNTER

THE CORINNE T. NETZER LOW FAT DIARY

THE DIETER'S CALORIE COUNTER

THE COMPLETE BOOK OF VITAMIN
& MINERAL COUNTS

CORINNE T. NETZER'S BIG BOOK OF
MIRACLE CURES

THE COMPLETE BOOK OF FOOD COUNTS
COOKBOOK SERIES:

100 LOW FAT SMALL MEAL AND SALAD RECIPES

100 LOW FAT VEGETABLE AND LEGUME RECIPES

100 LOW FAT SOUP AND STEW RECIPES

100 LOW FAT PASTA AND GRAIN RECIPES

100 LOW FAT FISH AND SHELLFISH RECIPES

100 LOW FAT CHICKEN AND TURKEY RECIPES

THE
CORINNE T. NETZER

CARBOHYDRATE
DIETER'S
DIARY

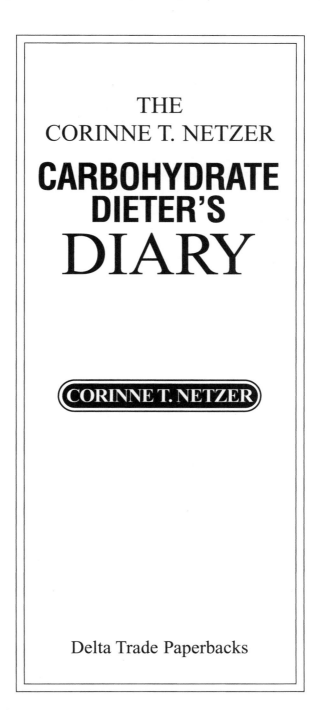

CORINNE T. NETZER

Delta Trade Paperbacks

THE CORINNE T. NETZER CARBOHYDRATE DIETER'S DIARY
A Delta Book

PUBLISHING HISTORY
Dell Trade Paperback edition published April 1999
Delta trade paperback edition / May 2006

Published by Bantam Dell
A Division of Random House, Inc.
New York, New York

All rights reserved
Copyright © 1999, 2006 by Corinne T. Netzer

Book design by Ellen Cipriano

Delta is a registered trademark of Random House, Inc., and
the colophon is a trademark of Random House, Inc.

ISBN-10: 0-440-50852-5
ISBN-13: 978-0-440-50852-6

Printed in the United States of America
Published simultaneously in Canada

www.bantamdell.com

RRH   11

THIS BOOK
BELONGS TO

_____

ADDRESS
....

CITY
....

STATE   ZIP CODE
....

HOME TELEPHONE
....

BUSINESS TELEPHONE
....

❖   ❖   ❖

IN CASE OF EMERGENCY NOTIFY:

NAME
....

ADDRESS
....

CITY
....

STATE   ZIP CODE
....

HOME TELEPHONE
....

BUSINESS TELEPHONE
....

GOALS

CURRENT WEIGHT ....

DESIRED WEIGHT ....

MEASUREMENTS ....

Bust/Chest: Current ....Desired ....

Waist: Current ....Desired ....

Hips: Current ....Desired ....

Thighs: Current ....Desired ....

EXERCISE

Current Daily Activities ....

....

....

....

....

....

....

....

....

Desired Daily Activities ....

....

....

....

....

....

....

....

....

DAY 1

DATE _____ WEIGHT _____

BREAKFAST   **CARBS**
. . . .
. . . .
. . . .
. . . .

LUNCH   . . . .
. . . .
. . . .
. . . .
. . . .

DINNER   . . . .
. . . .
. . . .
. . . .
. . . .
. . . .
. . . .
. . . .

SNACKS   . . . .
. . . .
. . . .
. . . .
. . . .

                                    TOTAL
                                    DAILY CARBOHYDRATES [   ]

COMMENTS
. . . .
. . . .
. . . .
. . . .

DAY 2

Desire is half the battle; commitment is the other half. Because you really want to stick to a diet and have started keeping this diary, you've won half the battle!

DATE _____ WEIGHT _____

BREAKFAST	CARBS
....	....
....	....
....	....
....	....

LUNCH	
....	....
....	....
....	....
....	....
....	....

DINNER	
....	....
....	....
....	....
....	....
....	....
....	....
....	....
....	....

SNACKS	
....	....
....	....
....	....
....	....

TOTAL
DAILY CARBOHYDRATES [   ]

COMMENTS
....
....
....
....

DAY 3

DATE   WEIGHT

BREAKFAST   **CARBS**
....
....
....
....

LUNCH   ....
....
....
....
....

DINNER   ....
....
....
....
....
....
....
....
....

SNACKS   ....
....
....
....
....

                        TOTAL
                        DAILY CARBOHYDRATES

COMMENTS
....
....
....
....

DAY 4

Diet one day at a time (it can be discouraging to think of giving up your favorite foods for weeks), and make a fresh resolution each morning that you'll stick to your diet.

DATE _____ WEIGHT _____

BREAKFAST	CARBS
....	....
....	....
....	....
....	....

LUNCH	
....	....
....	....
....	....
....	....

DINNER	
....	....
....	....
....	....
....	....
....	....
....	....
....	....

SNACKS	
....	....
....	....
....	....
....	....

TOTAL
DAILY CARBOHYDRATES [   ]

COMMENTS
....
....
....
....

DAY 5

DATE _____   WEIGHT _____

BREAKFAST	CARBS
....	....
....	....
....	....
....	....
....	....

LUNCH	
....	....
....	....
....	....
....	....
....	....

DINNER	
....	....
....	....
....	....
....	....
....	....
....	....
....	....
....	....

SNACKS	
....	....
....	....
....	....
....	....

TOTAL
DAILY CARBOHYDRATES [   ]

COMMENTS
....
....
....
....

DAY 6

Be aware that a "lite" or "dietary" version of a
food may be higher in carbohydrates. No-fat
sour cream, for example, contains four times
as many carbs as the full-fat.

DATE   WEIGHT

BREAKFAST   **CARBS**
....
....
....
....
....

LUNCH   ....
....
....
....
....

DINNER   ....
....
....
....
....
....
....
....

SNACKS   ....
....
....
....
....

                              TOTAL
                              DAILY CARBOHYDRATES [   ]

COMMENTS
....
....
....
....

DAY 7

DATE _____ WEIGHT _____

BREAKFAST .... **CARBS** ......
....
....
....
....

LUNCH ....
....
....
....
....

DINNER ....
....
....
....
....
....
....
....

SNACKS ....
....
....
....
....

TOTAL
DAILY CARBOHYDRATES [_____]

COMMENTS ....
....
....
....
....

WEEKLY
PROGRESS REPORT

DATE: From .... To ....

WEIGHT: ....

AVERAGE DAILY CARBOHYDRATE INTAKE* ....

MEASUREMENTS:

    Bust/Chest ....

    Waist ....

    Hips ....

    Thighs ....

EXERCISE:

    Day 1 ....

    Day 2 ....

    Day 3 ....

    Day 4 ....

    Day 5 ....

    Day 6 ....

    Day 7 ....

PLANS FOR NEXT WEEK:

....
....
....
....
....

*Add your daily carbohydrates for the week and divide by 7.

DAY 1

DATE _____ WEIGHT _____

BREAKFAST .... **CARBS**
....
....
....
....

LUNCH ....
....
....
....
....

DINNER ....
....
....
....
....
....
....
....

SNACKS ....
....
....
....

TOTAL
DAILY CARBOHYDRATES [   ]

COMMENTS ....
....
....
....

DAY 2

Spend your daily allotment of carbohydrates wisely. Instead of using it on sweets, choose fresh green vegetables and other low-carb, fiber-rich foods that are nutritious.

DATE .... WEIGHT ....

BREAKFAST .... **CARBS**

....

....

....

....

LUNCH ....

....

....

....

....

DINNER ....

....

....

....

....

....

....

....

SNACKS ....

....

....

....

....

TOTAL
DAILY CARBOHYDRATES

COMMENTS

....

....

....

DAY 3

DATE _____   WEIGHT _____

BREAKFAST .... **CARBS**
....
....
....
....

LUNCH ....
....
....
....
....

DINNER ....
....
....
....
....
....
....
....
....

SNACKS ....
....
....
....
....

TOTAL
DAILY CARBOHYDRATES [   ]

COMMENTS
....
....
....
....

DAY 4

Think of a better shape as well as
a thinner shape. When you're exercising,
concentrate on specific trouble spot(s): abdomen,
waist, hips, thighs, or buttocks.

DATE _____ WEIGHT _____

BREAKFAST   **CARBS**
....
....
....
....
....

LUNCH
....
....
....
....

DINNER
....
....
....
....
....
....
....

SNACKS
....
....
....
....

                              TOTAL
                              DAILY CARBOHYDRATES   [   ]

COMMENTS
....
....
....
....

DAY 5

DATE _____ WEIGHT _____

BREAKFAST   **CARBS**
....
....
....
....

LUNCH   ....
....
....
....
....

DINNER   ....
....
....
....
....
....
....
....

SNACKS   ....
....
....
....

                              TOTAL
                              DAILY CARBOHYDRATES   [   ]

COMMENTS
....
....
....
....

DAY 6

Writing everything down really works, but you must be honest. Record everything you eat and drink; otherwise you're only fooling yourself—and ruining your diet.

DATE _____ WEIGHT _____

BREAKFAST   **CARBS**

....

....

....

....

....

LUNCH

....

....

....

....

....

DINNER

....

....

....

....

....

....

....

....

SNACKS

....

....

....

....

....

                                    TOTAL
                                    DAILY CARBOHYDRATES   [   ]

COMMENTS

....

....

....

DAY 7

DATE _____ WEIGHT _____

BREAKFAST	**CARBS**
....	....
....	....
....	....
....	....
LUNCH	....
....	....
....	....
....	....
....	....
DINNER	....
....	....
....	....
....	....
....	....
....	....
....	....
SNACKS	....
....	....
....	....
....	....
....	....

TOTAL
DAILY CARBOHYDRATES [   ]

COMMENTS ....
....
....
....

WEEKLY
PROGRESS REPORT

DATE: From .... To ....

WEIGHT: ....

AVERAGE DAILY CARBOHYDRATE INTAKE* ....

MEASUREMENTS:

Bust/Chest ....

Waist ....

Hips ....

Thighs ....

EXERCISE:

Day 1 ....

....

Day 2 ....

....

Day 3 ....

....

Day 4 ....

....

Day 5 ....

....

Day 6 ....

....

Day 7 ....

....

PLANS FOR NEXT WEEK:

....

....

....

....

....

*Add your daily carbohydrates for the week and divide by 7.

DAY 1

DATE   WEIGHT

BREAKFAST   **CARBS**
....
....
....
....
....

LUNCH
....
....
....
....
....

DINNER
....
....
....
....
....
....
....
....

SNACKS
....
....
....
....
....

TOTAL
DAILY CARBOHYDRATES

COMMENTS
....
....
....
....

DAY 2

Even though some low-carb diets claim
it doesn't matter how much food you eat,
it's still a good idea to eat in moderation.
You won't lose as fast if you're overeating.

DATE   WEIGHT

BREAKFAST   **CARBS**
....
....
....
....

LUNCH
....
....
....
....

DINNER
....
....
....
....
....
....
....

SNACKS
....
....
....
....
....

                              TOTAL
                              DAILY CARBOHYDRATES [   ]

COMMENTS
....
....
....
....

DAY 3

DATE _____   WEIGHT _____

BREAKFAST . . . . **CARBS**

. . . .

. . . .

. . . .

. . . .

LUNCH . . . .

. . . .

. . . .

. . . .

. . . .

DINNER . . . .

. . . .

. . . .

. . . .

. . . .

. . . .

. . . .

. . . .

SNACKS . . . .

. . . .

. . . .

. . . .

. . . .

TOTAL
DAILY CARBOHYDRATES   [   ]

COMMENTS . . . .

. . . .

. . . .

. . . .

DAY 4

When you're craving a sweet snack, try
chewing on a thin slice of lemon or lime.
Some dieters claim it reduces the craving for
sweets, while others prefer a sour pickle.

DATE _____ WEIGHT _____

BREAKFAST   **CARBS**

....

....

....

....

LUNCH

....

....

....

....

....

DINNER

....

....

....

....

....

....

....

....

SNACKS

....

....

....

....

TOTAL
DAILY CARBOHYDRATES [   ]

COMMENTS

....

....

....

....

DAY 5

DATE _____   WEIGHT _____

BREAKFAST   CARBS

....

....

....

....

LUNCH   ....

....

....

....

....

DINNER   ....

....

....

....

....

....

....

....

SNACKS   ....

....

....

....

....

TOTAL
DAILY CARBOHYDRATES   [   ]

COMMENTS

....

....

....

....

DAY 6

Don't just assume that a food is low in
carbohydrates. If you're not certain, check
the carbohydrate content before you indulge
(see counter, pages 135-176).

DATE _____ WEIGHT _____

BREAKFAST .... **CARBS**

....

....

....

....

LUNCH ....

....

....

....

....

DINNER ....

....

....

....

....

....

....

....

SNACKS ....

....

....

....

....

TOTAL
DAILY CARBOHYDRATES

COMMENTS ....

....

....

....

DAY 7

DATE _____ WEIGHT _____

BREAKFAST   **CARBS**
....
....
....
....
....

LUNCH
....
....
....
....
....

DINNER
....
....
....
....
....
....
....
....
....

SNACKS
....
....
....
....

TOTAL
DAILY CARBOHYDRATES [   ]

COMMENTS
....
....
....
....

WEEKLY
PROGRESS REPORT

DATE: From .... To ....

WEIGHT: ....

AVERAGE DAILY CARBOHYDRATE INTAKE* ....

MEASUREMENTS:

Bust/Chest ....

Waist ....

Hips ....

Thighs ....

EXERCISE:

Day 1 ....

....

Day 2 ....

....

Day 3 ....

....

Day 4 ....

....

Day 5 ....

....

Day 6 ....

....

Day 7 ....

....

PLANS FOR NEXT WEEK:

....

....

....

....

....

*Add your daily carbohydrates for the week and divide by 7.

DAY 1

DATE _____ WEIGHT _____

BREAKFAST	CARBS
....	.....
....	.....
....	.....
....	.....

LUNCH	
....	.....
....	.....
....	.....
....	.....

DINNER	
....	.....
....	.....
....	.....
....	.....
....	.....
....	.....
....	.....

SNACKS	
....	.....
....	.....
....	.....
....	.....

TOTAL
DAILY CARBOHYDRATES [   ]

COMMENTS
....
....
....
....

DAY 2

Set up an object goal as well as a weight goal.
Instead of simply saying "I want to lose twenty
pounds by summer," you might add, "so I can be
slim enough to wear a bikini."

DATE _____ WEIGHT _____

BREAKFAST   **CARBS**

....
....
....
....

LUNCH

....
....
....
....

DINNER

....
....
....
....
....
....
....

SNACKS

....
....
....
....

TOTAL
DAILY CARBOHYDRATES [   ]

COMMENTS

....
....
....
....

DAY 3

DATE   WEIGHT

BREAKFAST   **CARBS**
....
....
....
....

LUNCH   ....
....
....
....
....
....

DINNER   ....
....
....
....
....
....
....
....
....

SNACKS   ....
....
....
....
....

TOTAL
DAILY CARBOHYDRATES

COMMENTS
....
....
....
....

DAY 4

Take up a hobby that will keep
your fingers busy. Try knitting or painting,
consider pottery, or surf the Web. Whatever it is,
reach for it instead of something to eat.

DATE _____ WEIGHT _____

BREAKFAST   **CARBS**

....

....

....

....

....

LUNCH

....

....

....

....

....

DINNER

....

....

....

....

....

....

....

....

....

SNACKS

....

....

....

....

TOTAL
DAILY CARBOHYDRATES [   ]

COMMENTS

....

....

....

....

DAY 5

DATE _____   WEIGHT _____

BREAKFAST   **CARBS**

....
....
....
....

LUNCH

....
....
....
....

DINNER

....
....
....
....
....
....
....

SNACKS

....
....
....
....
....

TOTAL
DAILY CARBOHYDRATES   [   ]

COMMENTS

....
....
....
....

DAY 6

Make a financial investment in your diet.
Whether it's membership in a gym or smaller-size
clothing, a dollar commitment is an
excellent incentive for staying on your diet.

DATE _____ WEIGHT _____

BREAKFAST   **CARBS**

....

....

....

....

LUNCH

....

....

....

....

DINNER

....

....

....

....

....

....

....

SNACKS

....

....

....

....

                      TOTAL
                      DAILY CARBOHYDRATES   [   ]

COMMENTS

....

....

....

....

DAY 7

DATE _____ WEIGHT _____

BREAKFAST .... **CARBS**

....

....

....

....

LUNCH ....

....

....

....

....

DINNER ....

....

....

....

....

....

....

....

SNACKS ....

....

....

....

....

TOTAL
DAILY CARBOHYDRATES [   ]

COMMENTS ....

....

....

....

WEEKLY
PROGRESS REPORT

DATE: From .... To ....

WEIGHT: ....

AVERAGE DAILY CARBOHYDRATE INTAKE* ....

MEASUREMENTS:

Bust/Chest ....

Waist ....

Hips ....

Thighs ....

EXERCISE:

Day 1 ....

....

Day 2 ....

....

Day 3 ....

....

Day 4 ....

....

Day 5 ....

....

Day 6 ....

....

Day 7 ....

....

PLANS FOR NEXT WEEK:

....
....
....
....
....

*Add your daily carbohydrates for the week and divide by 7.

DAY 1

DATE _____ WEIGHT _____

BREAKFAST   **CARBS**
....
....
....
....

LUNCH
....
....
....
....

DINNER
....
....
....
....
....
....
....

SNACKS
....
....
....
....

TOTAL
DAILY CARBOHYDRATES [   ]

COMMENTS
....
....
....
....

DAY 2

Be patient. Those extra pounds didn't
appear overnight and they won't go away
overnight. Dieting is hard work and you should
be prepared for occasional setbacks.

DATE _____   WEIGHT _____

BREAKFAST	CARBS
....	......
....	......
....	......
....	......
LUNCH	
....	......
....	......
....	......
....	......
DINNER	
....	......
....	......
....	......
....	......
....	......
....	......
....	......
....	......
SNACKS	
....	......
....	......
....	......
....	......

TOTAL
DAILY CARBOHYDRATES [   ]

COMMENTS
....
....
....
....

DAY 3

DATE _____ WEIGHT _____

BREAKFAST   **CARBS**
....
....
....
....

LUNCH
....
....
....
....

DINNER
....
....
....
....
....
....
....

SNACKS
....
....
....
....

TOTAL
DAILY CARBOHYDRATES [   ]

COMMENTS
....
....
....
....

DAY 4

Many dieters use their daily carbohydrate allotment on salads—they offer fiber, variety (add sprouts, asparagus, and other veggies), and a choice of rich dressings.

DATE _____ WEIGHT _____

BREAKFAST | **CARBS**
.... | ....
.... | ....
.... | ....
.... | ....
.... | ....

LUNCH
.... | ....
.... | ....
.... | ....
.... | ....
.... | ....

DINNER
.... | ....
.... | ....
.... | ....
.... | ....
.... | ....
.... | ....
.... | ....
.... | ....

SNACKS
.... | ....
.... | ....
.... | ....
.... | ....
.... | ....

TOTAL
DAILY CARBOHYDRATES [   ]

COMMENTS
....
....
....
....

DAY 5

DATE _____   WEIGHT _____

BREAKFAST	CARBS
....	....
....	....
....	....
....	....
LUNCH	
....	....
....	....
....	....
....	....
....	....
DINNER	
....	....
....	....
....	....
....	....
....	....
....	....
....	....
SNACKS	
....	....
....	....
....	....
....	....

TOTAL
DAILY CARBOHYDRATES [   ]

COMMENTS
....
....
....
....

DAY 6

Diet with your partner, lover, or friend.
Check on each other's progress as you provide
the support and encouragement that's
so essential while trying to lose weight.

DATE _____ WEIGHT _____

BREAKFAST	CARBS
....	.....
....	.....
....	.....
....	.....
LUNCH	.....
....	.....
....	.....
....	.....
....	.....
DINNER	.....
....	.....
....	.....
....	.....
....	.....
....	.....
....	.....
....	.....
SNACKS	.....
....	.....
....	.....
....	.....

TOTAL
DAILY CARBOHYDRATES [   ]

COMMENTS
....
....
....

DAY 7

DATE .... WEIGHT ....

BREAKFAST .... **CARBS**
....
....
....
....

LUNCH ....
....
....
....
....

DINNER ....
....
....
....
....
....
....
....
....

SNACKS ....
....
....
....

TOTAL
DAILY CARBOHYDRATES

COMMENTS ....
....
....
....

WEEKLY
PROGRESS REPORT

DATE: From .... To ....

WEIGHT: ....

AVERAGE DAILY CARBOHYDRATE INTAKE✿ ....

MEASUREMENTS:

Bust/Chest ....

Waist ....

Hips ....

Thighs ....

EXERCISE:

Day 1 ....
....

Day 2 ....
....

Day 3 ....
....

Day 4 ....
....

Day 5 ....
....

Day 6 ....
....

Day 7 ....
....

PLANS FOR NEXT WEEK:

....
....
....
....
....

✿Add your daily carbohydrates for the week and divide by 7.

DAY 1

DATE _____ WEIGHT _____

BREAKFAST .... **CARBS**
....
....
....
....

LUNCH ....
....
....
....
....

DINNER ....
....
....
....
....
....
....
....
....

SNACKS ....
....
....
....
....

TOTAL
DAILY CARBOHYDRATES [   ]

COMMENTS
....
....
....
....

DAY 2

If you have any unflattering, pre-diet photographs of yourself, display them where they will have immediate impact: on refrigerator, cupboard, and pantry doors.

DATE .... WEIGHT ....

BREAKFAST .... **CARBS**

....

....

....

....

LUNCH ....

....

....

....

....

DINNER ....

....

....

....

....

....

....

SNACKS ....

....

....

....

....

TOTAL
DAILY CARBOHYDRATES ☐

COMMENTS ....

....

....

....

DAY 3

DATE _____ WEIGHT _____

BREAKFAST .... **CARBS**
....
....
....
....

LUNCH ....
....
....
....
....

DINNER ....
....
....
....
....
....
....
....

SNACKS ....
....
....
....
....

TOTAL
DAILY CARBOHYDRATES [   ]

COMMENTS ....
....
....
....

DAY 4

Try making each meal an occasion. In dieting,
appearances do count. Setting a pretty
table with your best china, silver, and linens
will make you feel absolutely special.

DATE   WEIGHT

BREAKFAST   **CARBS**

....

....

....

....

....

LUNCH

....

....

....

....

DINNER

....

....

....

....

....

....

....

....

SNACKS

....

....

....

....

....

                              TOTAL
                              DAILY CARBOHYDRATES [   ]

COMMENTS

....

....

....

....

DAY 5

DATE   WEIGHT

BREAKFAST   **CARBS**
....
....
....
....

LUNCH
....
....
....
....
....

DINNER
....
....
....
....
....
....
....
....

SNACKS
....
....
....
....

TOTAL
DAILY CARBOHYDRATES

COMMENTS
....
....
....
....

DAY 6

Pinpoint the times (other than mealtimes)
when you're most tempted to go off your diet.
Plan something (walk, jog, make phone calls)
that keeps you away from food at that hour.

DATE _____ WEIGHT _____

BREAKFAST   **CARBS**
....
....
....
....
....

LUNCH
....
....
....
....
....

DINNER
....
....
....
....
....
....
....
....
....

SNACKS
....
....
....
....

                          TOTAL
                          DAILY CARBOHYDRATES   [   ]

COMMENTS
....
....
....
....

DAY 7

DATE .... WEIGHT ....

BREAKFAST .... **CARBS**
....
....
....
....

LUNCH ....
....
....
....
....
....

DINNER ....
....
....
....
....
....
....
....
....

SNACKS ....
....
....
....
....

TOTAL
DAILY CARBOHYDRATES

COMMENTS ....
....
....
....

WEEKLY
PROGRESS REPORT

DATE: From .... To ....

WEIGHT: ....

AVERAGE DAILY CARBOHYDRATE INTAKE＊ ....

MEASUREMENTS:

Bust/Chest ....

Waist ....

Hips ....

Thighs ....

EXERCISE:

Day 1 ....
....

Day 2 ....
....

Day 3 ....
....

Day 4 ....
....

Day 5 ....
....

Day 6 ....
....

Day 7 ....
....

PLANS FOR NEXT WEEK:

....
....
....
....
....

＊Add your daily carbohydrates for the week and divide by 7.

DAY 1

DATE _____ WEIGHT _____

BREAKFAST .... **CARBS**
....
....
....
....

LUNCH ....
....
....
....
....

DINNER ....
....
....
....
....
....
....
....
....

SNACKS ....
....
....
....
....

TOTAL
DAILY CARBOHYDRATES [   ]

COMMENTS
....
....
....
....

DAY 2

Do your food shopping after you have
eaten, never before. Traveling supermarket
aisles when you're hungry can lead to
buying all the wrong kinds of food.

DATE _____ WEIGHT _____

BREAKFAST	CARBS
....	....
....	....
....	....
....	....

LUNCH	
....	....
....	....
....	....
....	....
....	....

DINNER	
....	....
....	....
....	....
....	....
....	....
....	....
....	....
....	....

SNACKS	
....	....
....	....
....	....
....	....
....	....

TOTAL
DAILY CARBOHYDRATES [   ]

COMMENTS
....
....
....
....

DAY 3

DATE _____   WEIGHT _____

BREAKFAST . . . . **CARBS**

. . . .

. . . .

. . . .

. . . .

LUNCH . . . .

. . . .

. . . .

. . . .

. . . .

DINNER . . . .

. . . .

. . . .

. . . .

. . . .

. . . .

. . . .

. . . .

SNACKS . . . .

. . . .

. . . .

. . . .

. . . .

TOTAL
DAILY CARBOHYDRATES

COMMENTS

. . . .

. . . .

. . . .

. . . .

DAY 4

Try to fill your spare time. Sign up for
an evening course at your local school; do
volunteer work; get involved in a social,
political, community, or religious group.

DATE   WEIGHT

BREAKFAST   **CARBS**

....

....

....

....

LUNCH

....

....

....

....

....

DINNER

....

....

....

....

....

....

....

SNACKS

....

....

....

....

| | TOTAL
DAILY CARBOHYDRATES | |

COMMENTS

....

....

....

DAY 5

DATE _____   WEIGHT _____

BREAKFAST	**CARBS**
. . . .	. . . .
. . . .	. . . .
. . . .	. . . .
. . . .	. . . .

LUNCH	
. . . .	. . . .
. . . .	. . . .
. . . .	. . . .
. . . .	. . . .

DINNER	
. . . .	. . . .
. . . .	. . . .
. . . .	. . . .
. . . .	. . . .
. . . .	. . . .
. . . .	. . . .

SNACKS	
. . . .	. . . .
. . . .	. . . .
. . . .	. . . .
. . . .	. . . .

TOTAL
DAILY CARBOHYDRATES [   ]

COMMENTS
. . . .
. . . .
. . . .
. . . .

DAY 6

A low-carbohydrate diet doesn't have to be a high-fat diet. Make an effort to limit fat intake—remove skin from chicken, fat from steak, stick to lean luncheon meats.

DATE _____ WEIGHT _____

BREAKFAST   **CARBS**

....
....
....
....

LUNCH

....
....
....
....

DINNER

....
....
....
....
....
....
....
....

SNACKS

....
....
....
....

TOTAL
DAILY CARBOHYDRATES [   ]

COMMENTS

....
....
....
....

DAY 7

DATE   WEIGHT

BREAKFAST   **CARBS**

....

....

....

....

....

LUNCH

....

....

....

....

....

DINNER

....

....

....

....

....

....

....

....

SNACKS

....

....

....

....

TOTAL
DAILY CARBOHYDRATES

COMMENTS

....

....

....

....

WEEKLY
PROGRESS REPORT

DATE: From .... To ....

WEIGHT: ....

AVERAGE DAILY CARBOHYDRATE INTAKE* ....

MEASUREMENTS:

    Bust/Chest ....

    Waist ....

    Hips ....

    Thighs ....

EXERCISE:

    Day 1 ....
    ....

    Day 2 ....
    ....

    Day 3 ....
    ....

    Day 4 ....
    ....

    Day 5 ....
    ....

    Day 6 ....
    ....

    Day 7 ....
    ....

PLANS FOR NEXT WEEK:

....
....
....
....
....

*Add your daily carbohydrates for the week and divide by 7.

DAY 1

DATE _____ WEIGHT _____

BREAKFAST	CARBS
....	....
....	....
....	....
....	....
LUNCH	....
....	....
....	....
....	....
....	....
....	....
DINNER	....
....	....
....	....
....	....
....	....
....	....
....	....
....	....
SNACKS	....
....	....
....	....
....	....
....	....

TOTAL
DAILY CARBOHYDRATES [   ]

COMMENTS ....
....
....
....

DAY 2

Prepare a "paper-bag" lunch to take to
work. You'll find it far easier to meet
your diet quotas by deciding on lunches for
yourself—and you'll save money as well.

DATE _____ WEIGHT _____

BREAKFAST	CARBS
....	....
....	....
....	....
....	....
LUNCH	....
....	....
....	....
....	....
....	....
DINNER	....
....	....
....	....
....	....
....	....
....	....
....	....
....	....
SNACKS	....
....	....
....	....
....	....
....	....

TOTAL
DAILY CARBOHYDRATES [   ]

COMMENTS
....
....
....
....

DAY 3

DATE _____   WEIGHT _____

BREAKFAST   **CARBS**
....
....
....
....
....

LUNCH
....
....
....
....
....

DINNER
....
....
....
....
....
....
....
....

SNACKS
....
....
....
....

                                TOTAL
                                DAILY CARBOHYDRATES   [   ]

COMMENTS
....
....
....
....

DAY 4

Drink lots of water throughout the day.
Water fills the stomach, decreases the appetite,
facilitates excretion of waste materials,
and cleanses the system of impurities.

DATE   WEIGHT

BREAKFAST   **CARBS**

....

....

....

....

LUNCH   ....

....

....

....

....

DINNER

....

....

....

....

....

....

....

SNACKS   ....

....

....

....

....

TOTAL
DAILY CARBOHYDRATES

COMMENTS

....

....

....

....

DAY 5

DATE   WEIGHT

BREAKFAST   **CARBS**
....
....
....
....

LUNCH
....
....
....
....
....

DINNER
....
....
....
....
....
....
....
....

SNACKS
....
....
....
....

                              TOTAL
                              DAILY CARBOHYDRATES

COMMENTS
....
....
....
....

DAY 6

Seafood is a good diet choice and comes
in many tastes and textures. Experiment with
different fish and cooking methods: baking,
broiling, grilling, poaching, and sautéing.

DATE .... WEIGHT ....

BREAKFAST .... **CARBS**

....
....
....
....

LUNCH ....

....
....
....
....

DINNER ....

....
....
....
....
....
....
....

SNACKS ....

....
....
....
....

TOTAL
DAILY CARBOHYDRATES

COMMENTS

....
....
....
....

DAY 7

DATE _____   WEIGHT _____

BREAKFAST   **CARBS**
....
....
....
....

LUNCH
....
....
....
....

DINNER
....
....
....
....
....
....
....

SNACKS
....
....
....
....

TOTAL
DAILY CARBOHYDRATES [   ]

COMMENTS
....
....
....
....

WEEKLY PROGRESS REPORT

DATE: From .... To ....

WEIGHT: ....

AVERAGE DAILY CARBOHYDRATE INTAKE* ....

MEASUREMENTS:

Bust/Chest ....

Waist ....

Hips ....

Thighs ....

EXERCISE:

Day 1 ....

....

Day 2 ....

....

Day 3 ....

....

Day 4 ....

....

Day 5 ....

....

Day 6 ....

....

Day 7 ....

....

PLANS FOR NEXT WEEK:

....

....

....

....

....

*Add your daily carbohydrates for the week and divide by 7.

DAY 1

DATE .... WEIGHT ....

BREAKFAST   **CARBS**

....

....

....

....

LUNCH

....

....

....

....

....

DINNER

....

....

....

....

....

....

....

SNACKS

....

....

....

....

TOTAL
DAILY CARBOHYDRATES

COMMENTS

....

....

....

....

DAY 2

Carry low-carb snacks with you for those
times you think you might want or need
some. Cashews, macadamias, walnuts,
and other rich nuts are good choices.

DATE _____ WEIGHT _____

BREAKFAST   **CARBS**
....
....
....
....
....

LUNCH   ....
....
....
....
....
....

DINNER   ....
....
....
....
....
....
....
....
....

SNACKS   ....
....
....
....
....

                          TOTAL
                          DAILY CARBOHYDRATES   [   ]

COMMENTS
....
....
....
....

DAY 3

DATE   WEIGHT

BREAKFAST   **CARBS**

....

....

....

....

LUNCH   ....

....

....

....

....

DINNER   ....

....

....

....

....

....

....

....

SNACKS   ....

....

....

....

....

TOTAL
DAILY CARBOHYDRATES

COMMENTS

....

....

....

....

DAY 4

Try this instead of a bedtime snack: Before
going to the kitchen, stop and brush your teeth
thoroughly, then rinse with a mouthwash.
That craving will probably disappear.

DATE   WEIGHT

BREAKFAST   **CARBS**

....
....
....
....

LUNCH

....
....
....
....

DINNER

....
....
....
....
....
....
....

SNACKS

....
....
....
....

| | TOTAL | |
| | DAILY CARBOHYDRATES | |

COMMENTS

....
....
....

DAY 5

DATE .... WEIGHT ....

BREAKFAST .... **CARBS**

....

....

....

....

LUNCH ....

....

....

....

....

DINNER ....

....

....

....

....

....

....

....

SNACKS ....

....

....

....

....

TOTAL
DAILY CARBOHYDRATES

COMMENTS

....

....

....

....

DAY 6

Diet for the long term. It's faulty reasoning
to believe that if you've been "bad" for a day
your diet is over. Start again. That's why this
book has Weekly Progress Reports.

DATE _____ WEIGHT _____

BREAKFAST   **CARBS**
....
....
....
....
....

LUNCH
....
....
....
....
....

DINNER
....
....
....
....
....
....
....
....

SNACKS
....
....
....
....

                          TOTAL
                          DAILY CARBOHYDRATES   [   ]

COMMENTS
....
....
....

76

DAY 7

DATE .... WEIGHT ....

BREAKFAST	**CARBS**
....	....
....	....
....	....
....	....
LUNCH	....
....	....
....	....
....	....
....	....
DINNER	....
....	....
....	....
....	....
....	....
....	....
....	....
....	....
SNACKS	....
....	....
....	....
....	....
....	....

TOTAL
DAILY CARBOHYDRATES [   ]

COMMENTS
....
....
....
....

WEEKLY
PROGRESS REPORT

DATE: From .... To ....

WEIGHT: ....

AVERAGE DAILY CARBOHYDRATE INTAKE* ....

MEASUREMENTS:

   Bust/Chest ....

   Waist ....

   Hips ....

   Thighs ....

EXERCISE:

   Day 1 ....

   ....

   Day 2 ....

   ....

   Day 3 ....

   ....

   Day 4 ....

   ....

   Day 5 ....

   ....

   Day 6 ....

   ....

   Day 7 ....

   ....

PLANS FOR NEXT WEEK:

....

....

....

....

....

*Add your daily carbohydrates for the week and divide by 7.

DAY 1

DATE   WEIGHT

BREAKFAST .... **CARBS**
....
....
....
....

LUNCH ....
....
....
....
....

DINNER ....
....
....
....
....
....
....
....
....

SNACKS ....
....
....
....
....

TOTAL
DAILY CARBOHYDRATES

COMMENTS ....
....
....
....
....

DAY 2

Think food through. When you crave a
forbidden food, imagine your feelings
after you've eaten it and focus on the fact
that it isn't worth the remorse you'll feel.

DATE .... WEIGHT ....

BREAKFAST   **CARBS**
....
....
....
....
....

LUNCH
....
....
....
....
....

DINNER
....
....
....
....
....
....
....
....

SNACKS
....
....
....
....
....

TOTAL
DAILY CARBOHYDRATES [   ]

COMMENTS
....
....
....
....

DAY 3

DATE _____   WEIGHT _____

BREAKFAST   **CARBS**
....
....
....
....

LUNCH
....
....
....
....

DINNER
....
....
....
....
....
....
....

SNACKS
....
....
....
....

TOTAL
DAILY CARBOHYDRATES   [   ]

COMMENTS
....
....
....
....

DAY 4

Stock up on a supply of diet-permitted
snack foods that you truly enjoy. That way,
whenever you get the urge to snack,
you'll have a satisfying tidbit on hand.

DATE _____ WEIGHT _____

BREAKFAST   **CARBS**

....
....
....
....

LUNCH   ....
....
....
....
....

DINNER   ....
....
....
....
....
....
....
....

SNACKS   ....
....
....
....
....

                              TOTAL
                              DAILY CARBOHYDRATES   [   ]

COMMENTS
....
....
....
....

DAY 5

DATE _____ WEIGHT _____

BREAKFAST	CARBS
....	....
....	....
....	....
....	....
LUNCH	....
....	....
....	....
....	....
....	....
....	....
DINNER	....
....	....
....	....
....	....
....	....
....	....
....	....
....	....
SNACKS	....
....	....
....	....
....	....
....	....

TOTAL
DAILY CARBOHYDRATES [   ]

COMMENTS
....
....
....
....

DAY 6

Think positively. Instead of dwelling on
how overweight you are, focus on how
slim and well proportioned you'll look when
you reach your diet goal.

DATE   WEIGHT

BREAKFAST   **CARBS**

....

....

....

....

LUNCH   ....

....

....

....

....

DINNER   ....

....

....

....

....

....

....

....

SNACKS   ....

....

....

....

....

TOTAL
DAILY CARBOHYDRATES

COMMENTS

....

....

....

....

DAY 7

DATE _____ WEIGHT _____

BREAKFAST   **CARBS**
....
....
....
....
....

LUNCH   ....
....
....
....
....
....

DINNER   ....
....
....
....
....
....
....
....
....

SNACKS   ....
....
....
....
....

                                    TOTAL
                                    DAILY CARBOHYDRATES [____]

COMMENTS ....
....
....
....

WEEKLY
PROGRESS REPORT

DATE: From .... To ....

WEIGHT: ....

AVERAGE DAILY CARBOHYDRATE INTAKE* ....

MEASUREMENTS:

    Bust/Chest ....

    Waist ....

    Hips ....

    Thighs ....

EXERCISE:

    Day 1 ....
    ....

    Day 2 ....
    ....

    Day 3 ....
    ....

    Day 4 ....
    ....

    Day 5 ....
    ....

    Day 6 ....
    ....

    Day 7 ....
    ....

PLANS FOR NEXT WEEK:

....
....
....
....
....

*Add your daily carbohydrates for the week and divide by 7.

DAY 1

DATE _____ WEIGHT _____

BREAKFAST	CARBS
....	....
....	....
....	....
....	....
LUNCH	
....	....
....	....
....	....
....	....
DINNER	
....	....
....	....
....	....
....	....
....	....
....	....
....	....
SNACKS	
....	....
....	....
....	....
....	....

TOTAL
DAILY CARBOHYDRATES [ ]

COMMENTS
....
....
....
....

DAY 2

Don't be discouraged by "diet plateaus,"
when your weight stays at the same level no
matter how conscientious you've been.
Every dieter has them, and they do pass.

DATE   WEIGHT

BREAKFAST   **CARBS**
....
....
....
....
....

LUNCH   ....
....
....
....
....
....

DINNER   ....
....
....
....
....
....
....
....

SNACKS   ....
....
....
....
....

                              TOTAL
                              DAILY CARBOHYDRATES

COMMENTS
....
....
....
....

DAY 3

DATE _____   WEIGHT _____

BREAKFAST ....   **CARBS**
....
....
....
....

LUNCH ....
....
....
....
....

DINNER ....
....
....
....
....
....
....
....

SNACKS ....
....
....
....
....

TOTAL
DAILY CARBOHYDRATES [   ]

COMMENTS
....
....
....
....

DAY 4

Use herbs and spices to flavor foods and add zest to bland meals. Experiment with a variety of exotic herbs and spices, but be sparing because they go a long way.

DATE _____ WEIGHT _____

BREAKFAST	CARBS
....	....
....	....
....	....
....	....
LUNCH	
....	....
....	....
....	....
....	....
....	....
DINNER	
....	....
....	....
....	....
....	....
....	....
....	....
....	....
....	....
SNACKS	
....	....
....	....
....	....
....	....

TOTAL
DAILY CARBOHYDRATES [   ]

COMMENTS
....
....
....
....

DAY 5

DATE   WEIGHT

BREAKFAST   **CARBS**
....
....
....
....

LUNCH   ....
....
....
....
....

DINNER   ....
....
....
....
....
....
....
....

SNACKS   ....
....
....
....
....

                              TOTAL
                              DAILY CARBOHYDRATES   [   ]

COMMENTS
....
....
....
....

DAY 6

Keep tempting foods out of reach. Even the
strongest-willed dieter has a blue day when a
chocolate bar or a bag of potato chips would
provide emotional comfort.

DATE _____ WEIGHT _____

BREAKFAST	CARBS

LUNCH	

DINNER	

SNACKS	

TOTAL
DAILY CARBOHYDRATES [   ]

COMMENTS

DAY 7

DATE _____   WEIGHT _____

BREAKFAST .... **CARBS**
....
....
....
....

LUNCH ....
....
....
....
....

DINNER ....
....
....
....
....
....
....
....

SNACKS ....
....
....
....

TOTAL
DAILY CARBOHYDRATES [   ]

COMMENTS ....
....
....
....

WEEKLY
PROGRESS REPORT

DATE: From .... To ....

WEIGHT: ....

AVERAGE DAILY CARBOHYDRATE INTAKE* ....

MEASUREMENTS:

Bust/Chest ....

Waist ....

Hips ....

Thighs ....

EXERCISE:

Day 1 ....

....

Day 2 ....

....

Day 3 ....

....

Day 4 ....

....

Day 5 ....

....

Day 6 ....

....

Day 7 ....

....

PLANS FOR NEXT WEEK:

....

....

....

....

....

*Add your daily carbohydrates for the week and divide by 7.

DAY 1

DATE _____   WEIGHT _____

BREAKFAST   **CARBS**
....
....
....
....

LUNCH   ....
....
....
....
....

DINNER   ....
....
....
....
....
....
....
....

SNACKS   ....
....
....
....
....

                                    TOTAL
                                    DAILY CARBOHYDRATES   [   ]

COMMENTS
....
....
....
....

DAY 2

When eating out, tell the waiter not to bring
bread and to hold the potatoes. Order turkey
without the gravy and stuffing, and indulge
your crouton-free salad with a rich dressing.

DATE _____ WEIGHT _____

BREAKFAST	CARBS
....	....
....	....
....	....
....	....

LUNCH	
....	....
....	....
....	....
....	....

DINNER	
....	....
....	....
....	....
....	....
....	....
....	....
....	....

SNACKS	
....	....
....	....
....	....
....	....

TOTAL
DAILY CARBOHYDRATES [   ]

COMMENTS
....
....
....
....

DAY 3

DATE _____   WEIGHT _____

BREAKFAST   **CARBS**

....

....

....

....

LUNCH

....

....

....

....

DINNER

....

....

....

....

....

....

....

SNACKS

....

....

....

....

TOTAL
DAILY CARBOHYDRATES   [   ]

COMMENTS

....

....

....

....

DAY 4

Is a sandwich your usual lunch? Make
yours without the bread. Use sliced luncheon
meats and cheese; spread with mayonnaise
and a bit of mustard and roll up or fold over.

DATE _____ WEIGHT _____

BREAKFAST .... **CARBS**

....

....

....

....

LUNCH ....

....

....

....

....

DINNER ....

....

....

....

....

....

....

....

....

SNACKS ....

....

....

....

....

TOTAL
DAILY CARBOHYDRATES [   ]

COMMENTS ....

....

....

....

DAY 5

DATE _____   WEIGHT _____

BREAKFAST   **CARBS**

....
....
....
....

LUNCH

....
....
....
....

DINNER

....
....
....
....
....
....
....

SNACKS

....
....
....
....

TOTAL
DAILY CARBOHYDRATES   [   ]

COMMENTS

....
....
....
....

DAY 6

Reward yourself. At the end of each week
or month of successful dieting, treat yourself
to a new scarf, a video or compact disc, a
book—but don't reward yourself with food.

DATE   WEIGHT

BREAKFAST   **CARBS**

....
....
....
....

LUNCH

....
....
....
....

DINNER

....
....
....
....
....
....
....

SNACKS

....
....
....
....

                        TOTAL
                        DAILY CARBOHYDRATES [   ]

COMMENTS
....
....
....
....

DAY 7

DATE _____ WEIGHT _____

BREAKFAST .... **CARBS**
....
....
....
....

LUNCH ....
....
....
....
....

DINNER ....
....
....
....
....
....
....
....

SNACKS ....
....
....
....

TOTAL
DAILY CARBOHYDRATES [   ]

COMMENTS ....
....
....
....

WEEKLY PROGRESS REPORT

DATE: From .... To ....

WEIGHT: ....

AVERAGE DAILY CARBOHYDRATE INTAKE✲ ....

MEASUREMENTS:

    Bust/Chest ....

    Waist ....

    Hips ....

    Thighs ....

EXERCISE:

    Day 1

    Day 2

    Day 3

    Day 4

    Day 5

    Day 6

    Day 7

PLANS FOR NEXT WEEK:

✲Add your daily carbohydrates for the week and divide by 7.

DAY 1

DATE .... WEIGHT ....

BREAKFAST .... **CARBS** ....
....
....
....
....

LUNCH ....
....
....
....
....

DINNER ....
....
....
....
....
....
....
....

SNACKS ....
....
....
....

TOTAL
DAILY CARBOHYDRATES

COMMENTS ....
....
....
....

DAY 2

If you should get depressed or discouraged over dieting, imagine all the new activities and pleasures your new appearance will allow, including fashionable clothing.

DATE _____ WEIGHT _____

BREAKFAST   **CARBS**
....
....
....
....
....

LUNCH
....
....
....
....
....

DINNER
....
....
....
....
....
....
....
....

SNACKS
....
....
....
....

                              TOTAL
                              DAILY CARBOHYDRATES [   ]

COMMENTS
....
....
....

DAY 3

DATE _____   WEIGHT _____

BREAKFAST .... **CARBS**

....

....

....

....

LUNCH ....

....

....

....

....

DINNER ....

....

....

....

....

....

....

....

SNACKS ....

....

....

....

TOTAL
DAILY CARBOHYDRATES [_____]

COMMENTS ....

....

....

....

....

DAY 4

Walking, skipping rope, and climbing stairs are
terrific exercises; they're also free and readily
available. (Be sure to check with your doctor
before starting any exercise program.)

DATE _____ WEIGHT _____

BREAKFAST   **CARBS**
....
....
....
....
....

LUNCH
....
....
....
....
....

DINNER
....
....
....
....
....
....
....
....

SNACKS
....
....
....
....

                              TOTAL
                              DAILY CARBOHYDRATES [   ]

COMMENTS
....
....
....

DAY 5

DATE _____ WEIGHT _____

BREAKFAST .... **CARBS**
....
....
....
....

LUNCH ....
....
....
....
....

DINNER ....
....
....
....
....
....
....
....

SNACKS ....
....
....
....

TOTAL
DAILY CARBOHYDRATES

COMMENTS ....
....
....
....

DAY 6

When you want a snack, reach for tasty,
low-carb cheese. Wrap up some slices of
your favorite kind and bring them along
to the movies in place of popcorn.

DATE   WEIGHT

BREAKFAST   **CARBS**

....

....

....

....

LUNCH

....

....

....

....

DINNER

....

....

....

....

....

....

....

....

SNACKS

....

....

....

....

TOTAL
DAILY CARBOHYDRATES

COMMENTS

....

....

....

DAY 7

DATE _____   WEIGHT _____

BREAKFAST   CARBS

....

....

....

....

LUNCH

....

....

....

....

DINNER

....

....

....

....

....

....

....

SNACKS

....

....

....

....

TOTAL
DAILY CARBOHYDRATES [   ]

COMMENTS

....

....

....

....

WEEKLY PROGRESS REPORT

DATE: From .... To ....

WEIGHT: ....

AVERAGE DAILY CARBOHYDRATE INTAKE* ....

MEASUREMENTS:

Bust/Chest ....

Waist ....

Hips ....

Thighs ....

EXERCISE:

Day 1 ....

....

Day 2 ....

....

Day 3 ....

....

Day 4 ....

....

Day 5 ....

....

Day 6 ....

....

Day 7 ....

....

PLANS FOR NEXT WEEK:

....
....
....
....
....

*Add your daily carbohydrates for the week and divide by 7.

DAY 1

DATE _____ WEIGHT _____

BREAKFAST . . . . **CARBS**

. . . .

. . . .

. . . .

. . . .

LUNCH

. . . .

. . . .

. . . .

. . . .

DINNER

. . . .

. . . .

. . . .

. . . .

. . . .

. . . .

SNACKS

. . . .

. . . .

. . . .

. . . .

TOTAL
DAILY CARBOHYDRATES [   ]

COMMENTS . . . .

. . . .

. . . .

. . . .

DAY 2

Eat a variety of meat, fish, and poultry, and
experiment with ways to cook and season them.
Boredom can be an enemy of progress and you
may find yourself breaking your diet.

DATE .... WEIGHT ....

BREAKFAST .... **CARBS**

....

....

....

....

LUNCH ....

....

....

....

....

DINNER ....

....

....

....

....

....

....

....

SNACKS ....

....

....

....

....

TOTAL
DAILY CARBOHYDRATES [   ]

COMMENTS ....

....

....

....

DAY 3

DATE _____ WEIGHT _____

BREAKFAST   **CARBS**

....

....

....

....

LUNCH

....

....

....

....

DINNER

....

....

....

....

....

....

....

SNACKS

....

....

....

....

TOTAL
DAILY CARBOHYDRATES   [_____]

COMMENTS

....

....

....

....

DAY 4

When you go out to dinner at overly generous
restaurants, consider sharing a meal. Take the
protein portion and give the high-carbohydrate
foods to your non-dieting friend.

DATE _____ WEIGHT _____

BREAKFAST .... **CARBS**
....
....
....
....

LUNCH ....
....
....
....
....

DINNER ....
....
....
....
....
....
....
....

SNACKS ....
....
....
....
....

                                    TOTAL
                                    DAILY CARBOHYDRATES [   ]

COMMENTS ....
....
....
....

DAY 5

DATE .... WEIGHT ....

BREAKFAST .... **CARBS**

....

....

....

....

LUNCH ....

....

....

....

....

DINNER ....

....

....

....

....

....

....

....

SNACKS ....

....

....

....

....

	TOTAL DAILY CARBOHYDRATES	

COMMENTS ....

....

....

....

DAY 6

If you're a snacker, try eating only when
you are really hungry. Concentrate on what
you're eating—and stop eating the minute
you feel that your hunger has been satisfied.

DATE   WEIGHT

BREAKFAST   **CARBS**

....

....

....

....

LUNCH

....

....

....

....

DINNER

....

....

....

....

....

....

....

SNACKS

....

....

....

....

TOTAL
DAILY CARBOHYDRATES

COMMENTS

....

....

....

....

DAY 7

DATE _____ WEIGHT _____

BREAKFAST   CARBS

....
....
....
....

LUNCH

....
....
....
....

DINNER

....
....
....
....
....
....
....
....

SNACKS

....
....
....
....

TOTAL
DAILY CARBOHYDRATES [   ]

COMMENTS

....
....
....
....

WEEKLY
PROGRESS REPORT

DATE: From .... To ....

WEIGHT: ....

AVERAGE DAILY CARBOHYDRATE INTAKE* ....

MEASUREMENTS:

    Bust/Chest ....

    Waist ....

    Hips ....

    Thighs ....

EXERCISE:

    Day 1 ....

    ....

    Day 2 ....

    ....

    Day 3 ....

    ....

    Day 4 ....

    ....

    Day 5 ....

    ....

    Day 6 ....

    ....

    Day 7 ....

    ....

PLANS FOR NEXT WEEK:

....

....

....

....

....

*Add your daily carbohydrates for the week and divide by 7.

DAY 1

DATE .... WEIGHT ....

BREAKFAST .... **CARBS**
....
....
....
....

LUNCH ....
....
....
....
....

DINNER ....
....
....
....
....
....
....
....

SNACKS ....
....
....
....
....

TOTAL
DAILY CARBOHYDRATES

COMMENTS ....
....
....
....
....

DAY 2

Exercise to easy-listening music. It's been
proven that the slower beat actually makes
people exercise longer and stronger because
they think their workouts are easier.

DATE _____ WEIGHT _____

BREAKFAST   **CARBS**

....
....
....
....

LUNCH

....
....
....
....
....

DINNER

....
....
....
....
....
....
....
....

SNACKS

....
....
....
....

TOTAL
DAILY CARBOHYDRATES [   ]

COMMENTS

....
....
....
....

DAY 3

DATE _____ WEIGHT _____

BREAKFAST .... **CARBS**
....
....
....
....

LUNCH ....
....
....
....
....

DINNER ....
....
....
....
....
....
....
....
....

SNACKS ....
....
....
....
....

TOTAL
DAILY CARBOHYDRATES [   ]

COMMENTS ....
....
....
....

DAY 4

Make a shopping list and try to stick to
it. This way you're more likely to stock up
on permitted foods and avoid any "impulse
foods" that markets know are hard to resist.

DATE   WEIGHT

BREAKFAST   **CARBS**

....

....

....

....

LUNCH

....

....

....

....

....

DINNER

....

....

....

....

....

....

....

....

....

SNACKS

....

....

....

....

TOTAL
DAILY CARBOHYDRATES

COMMENTS

....

....

....

DAY 5

DATE _____   WEIGHT _____

BREAKFAST ....   **CARBS**
....
....
....
....

LUNCH ....
....
....
....
....

DINNER ....
....
....
....
....
....
....
....
....

SNACKS ....
....
....
....
....

TOTAL
DAILY CARBOHYDRATES [   ]

COMMENTS ....
....
....
....
....

DAY 6

Cocktail parties with high-carb foods
can be a real challenge to your willpower.
Look for smoked salmon, tiny meatballs,
pâté, and cheese without the crackers.

DATE _____ WEIGHT _____

BREAKFAST .... **CARBS**

....

....

....

....

LUNCH ....

....

....

....

....

DINNER ....

....

....

....

....

....

....

....

....

SNACKS ....

....

....

....

TOTAL
DAILY CARBOHYDRATES [   ]

COMMENTS ....

....

....

....

DAY 7

DATE _____   WEIGHT _____

BREAKFAST   CARBS
....
....
....
....

LUNCH   ....
....
....
....
....

DINNER   ....
....
....
....
....
....
....
....

SNACKS   ....
....
....
....

                              TOTAL
                              DAILY CARBOHYDRATES   [   ]

COMMENTS
....
....
....
....

WEEKLY
PROGRESS REPORT

DATE: From .... To ....

WEIGHT: ....

AVERAGE DAILY CARBOHYDRATE INTAKE✲ ....

MEASUREMENTS:

Bust/Chest ....

Waist ....

Hips ....

Thighs ....

EXERCISE:

Day 1 ....
....

Day 2 ....
....

Day 3 ....
....

Day 4 ....
....

Day 5 ....
....

Day 6 ....
....

Day 7 ....
....

PLANS FOR NEXT WEEK:

....
....
....
....
....

✲Add your daily carbohydrates for the week and divide by 7.

DAY 1

DATE _____   WEIGHT _____

BREAKFAST   **CARBS**
....
....
....
....
....

LUNCH   ....
....
....
....
....
....

DINNER   ....
....
....
....
....
....
....
....
....

SNACKS   ....
....
....
....
....

                          TOTAL
                          DAILY CARBOHYDRATES   [   ]

COMMENTS
....
....
....
....

DAY 2

Remove the word "failure" from your
vocabulary. If you have an occasional slip
you haven't "failed," you've just had a slip.
Resolve to be more careful in the future.

DATE _____ WEIGHT _____

BREAKFAST   **CARBS**

....

....

....

....

LUNCH ....

....

....

....

....

DINNER ....

....

....

....

....

....

....

....

SNACKS ....

....

....

....

TOTAL
DAILY CARBOHYDRATES [   ]

COMMENTS

....

....

....

DAY 3

DATE _____ WEIGHT _____

BREAKFAST   **CARBS**
....
....
....
....
....

LUNCH   ....
....
....
....
....

DINNER   ....
....
....
....
....
....
....
....

SNACKS   ....
....
....
....
....

                              TOTAL
                              DAILY CARBOHYDRATES [   ]

COMMENTS
....
....
....
....

DAY 4

Altering your eating habits begs for support
and encouragement. Surround yourself with
like-minded friends and plan activities
together, such as sports, exercise, shopping.

DATE _____ WEIGHT _____

BREAKFAST   **CARBS**
....
....
....
....
....

LUNCH   ....
....
....
....
....
....

DINNER   ....
....
....
....
....
....
....
....
....

SNACKS   ....
....
....
....
....

                              TOTAL
                              DAILY CARBOHYDRATES [   ]

COMMENTS
....
....
....
....

DAY 5

DATE .... WEIGHT ....

BREAKFAST .... **CARBS**
....
....
....
....

LUNCH ....
....
....
....
....

DINNER ....
....
....
....
....
....
....
....

SNACKS ....
....
....
....

TOTAL
DAILY CARBOHYDRATES [   ]

COMMENTS ....
....
....
....

DAY 6

Congratulate yourself! You've made a
commitment to diet and exercise and you're
sticking to it. Just keep it up. This is one time
losing will make you a winner!

DATE _____ WEIGHT _____

BREAKFAST	CARBS
....	....
....	....
....	....
....	....
....	....

LUNCH	
....	....
....	....
....	....
....	....
....	....

DINNER	
....	....
....	....
....	....
....	....
....	....
....	....
....	....
....	....
....	....

SNACKS	
....	....
....	....
....	....
....	....

TOTAL
DAILY CARBOHYDRATES [   ]

COMMENTS
....
....
....

DAY 7

DATE _____   WEIGHT _____

BREAKFAST   **CARBS**
....
....
....
....

LUNCH
....
....
....
....
....

DINNER
....
....
....
....
....
....
....
....

SNACKS
....
....
....
....

TOTAL
DAILY CARBOHYDRATES [   ]

COMMENTS
....
....
....
....

WEEKLY
PROGRESS REPORT

DATE: From .... To ....

WEIGHT: ....

AVERAGE DAILY CARBOHYDRATE INTAKE* ....

MEASUREMENTS:

Bust/Chest ....

Waist ....

Hips ....

Thighs ....

EXERCISE:

Day 1 ....
....

Day 2 ....
....

Day 3 ....
....

Day 4 ....
....

Day 5 ....
....

Day 6 ....
....

Day 7 ....
....

PLANS FOR NEXT WEEK:

....
....
....
....
....

*Add your daily carbohydrates for the week and divide by 7.

DIETER'S
CARBOHYDRATE
GRAM COUNTER

ABBREVIATIONS & SYMBOLS

fl. .... fluid
" .... inch
diam. .... diameter
lb. .... pound
oz. .... ounce
pkt. .... packet
tbsp. .... tablespoon
tsp. .... teaspoon
< .... less than
*..... Prepared according to package
    directions

Abalone, raw, meat only, 4 oz. 6.8
Acerola, fresh, 10 fruits 3.7
Acerola juice, fresh, 8 fl. oz. 11.6
Acorn squash:
    baked, cubed, ½ cup 14.9
    boiled, mashed, ½ cup 10.8
Adzuki beans, boiled, ½ cup 28.5
Alfredo sauce, in jars, ¼ cup 3.0
Allspice, 1 tsp. 1.4
Almond, shelled:
    dried, 1 oz. 5.8
    dry-roasted, salted, 1 oz. 6.9
    honey-roasted, 1 oz. 7.9
    oil-roasted, salted, 1 oz. 4.5
    slivered, ¼ cup 6.9
Almond meal, 1 oz. 8.2
Amaranth, whole grain, 1 oz. 18.8
Amaranth leaves, boiled, drained, ½ cup 2.7
Anchovy, fresh or canned in oil 0
Anise seeds, 1 tsp. 1.1
Apple, fresh:
    raw, with peel, 2¾" apple 21.1
    raw, with peel, sliced, ½ cup 8.4
    raw, peeled, 2¾" apple 19.0
    raw, peeled, sliced, ½ cup 8.2
Apple, dried or dehydrated, ½ cup 28.2
Apple, frozen, ½ cup, unheated 10.7
Apple butter, 1 tbsp. 8.6
Apple juice, 8 fl. oz. 28.8
Applesauce:
    natural or unsweetened, ½ cup 13.8
    sweetened, ½ cup 25.5
Apricot, fresh:
    3 medium, 4 oz. 11.8
    pitted, sliced, ½ cup 9.2
Apricot, canned, halves:
    in juice, with liquid, ½ cup 15.1
    in light syrup, with liquid, ½ cup 20.9
    in heavy syrup, with liquid, ½ cup 27.7
Apricot, dried, sulfured, ½ cup 40.1
Apricot nectar, canned, 8 fl. oz. 36.1
Arctic char, without added ingredients 0
Arrowhead, boiled, drained, .4-oz. corm 1.9
Arrowroot, raw, sliced, ½ cup 8.0
Artichoke, globe, fresh:
    boiled, drained, 1 medium, 4.2 oz. edible 13.4

hearts, boiled, drained, ½ cup 9.4
Artichoke, canned, in water, hearts, 2 pieces 6.0
Artichoke, frozen, hearts, 9-oz. package 19.8
Artichoke, marinated, 1 oz. 2.0
Arugula, fresh, 10 leaves, 1 cup 7
Asparagus, fresh:
    boiled, 4 spears, ½"-diam. base 2.5
    boiled, drained, cuts, ½ cup 3.8
Asparagus, canned, ½ cup or 5 spears 3.0
Asparagus, frozen, 4 spears, 2 oz. 2.4
Avocado:
    all varieties, cubed, 1 cup 12.8
    California, pulp from 1 medium, 6.1 oz. 14.9
    California, pureed, ½ cup 9.9

B

carbohydrates

Bacon, pan-fried, 3 medium slices, 20 slices
    per lb. 1
Bacon, Canadian, unheated, 1-oz. slice 9
"Bacon" bits, imitation, 1 tbsp. 2.0
Bagel, plain, onion, sesame, or poppy seed, 2 oz. 32.2
Baked beans, canned, ½ cup:
    plain or vegetarian 26.1
    with franks 19.7
    with pork, in sweet sauce 26.5
    with pork, in tomato sauce 24.4
Baking mix, all purpose, ⅓ cup 26.0
Baking powder, 1 tsp. 1.1
Baking soda, 1 tsp. 0
Balsam pear, ½ cup:
    leafy tips, boiled, drained 2.0
    pods, boiled, drained, ½" pieces 2.7
Bamboo shoots, fresh, boiled, drained, ½ cup 1.2
Bamboo shoots, canned, drained, ½ cup 2.1
Banana (see also "Plantain"), fresh:
    1 medium, 8¾" long 26.7
    sliced, ½ cup 17.6
    red, 7¼" long 30.7
Banana, dried, dehydrated, ¼ cup 22.1
Banana chips, 1 oz. 16.6
Barbecue sauce, 2 tbsp. 9.0
Barley, pearled, cooked, ½ cup 22.2
Basil, fresh, 5 leaves or 1 tbsp. chopped 1
Basil, dried, crumbled, 1 tsp. 9
Bass, all varieties, without added ingredients 0
Bay leaf, dried, crumbled, 1 tsp. 3
Bean sprouts, fresh, 1 oz. 1.9

137

Beans, see specific listings

Beef, meat only, without added ingredients 0

Beef, corned, brisket, cooked, 4 oz. 5

Beef, corned, hash, canned, 1 cup 23.0

Beef, dried, cured, 1 oz. 4

Beef gravy, canned, ¼ cup 4.0

Beef jerky, chopped and formed, 1 oz. 4.1

Beefalo, meat only, without added ingredients 0

Beer:

    regular, 12 fl. oz. 13.2

    light, 12 fl. oz. 4.8

Beerwurst, pork and beef, 2 oz. 2.4

Beet, fresh:

    boiled, drained, 2 medium, 2" diam. 10.0

    boiled, drained, sliced, ½ cup 8.5

Beet, canned, ½ cup:

    whole or sliced, with liquid 8.3

    Harvard, with liquid 22.4

    pickled, with liquid 18.5

Beet greens, boiled, drained, 1" pieces, ½ cup 3.9

Berliner, pork and beef, 1 oz. 7

Biscuit, plain or buttermilk, 2-oz. piece 27.5

Black beans, dried, boiled, ½ cup 20.4

Black beans, canned, ½ cup 19.5

Blackberry, fresh, ½ cup 9.2

Black-eyed peas, dry, boiled, ½ cup 17.9

Black-eyed peas, canned, ½ cup 19.0

Blood sausage, 1 oz. 4

Blueberry, fresh, ½ cup 10.2

Blueberry, frozen, sweetened, ½ cup 25.2

Bluefish, without added ingredients 0

Bockwurst, raw, 1 oz. 1

Bok choy, see "Cabbage, Chinese"

Bologna:

    beef, 2 oz. 2.2

    beef and pork, 2 oz. 3.1

Bonito, meat only, raw, 4 oz. 5

Borage, boiled, drained, 4 oz. 4.0

Bouillon:

    beef flavor, 1 cube 6

    chicken flavor, 1 cube 1.1

Boysenberry, fresh, see "Blackberry"

Bran, see "Cereal" and specific grains

Bratwurst, pork, cooked, 2 oz. 1.2

Braunschweiger, pork, 2 oz. 2.0

Brazil nuts, shelled, 8 medium or 6 large, 1 oz. 3.6

Bread, 1-oz. slice, except as noted:

    French or Vienna 14.7

    Italian 14.2

mixed grain 13.1
oat bran 11.3
oatmeal 13.8
pita, white, 6½ diam., 2.25 oz. 33.4
pumpernickel 13.5
raisin 14.8
rice bran 12.3
rye 13.7
wheat 13.4
wheat bran or wheat germ 13.6
white 14.0
whole wheat 13.1
Bread crumbs, dry, ¼ cup or 1 oz. 19.5
Bread stick, plain, .5-oz. piece 7.0
Breadfruit, raw, ½ cup 29.8
Breadfruit seeds, roasted, shelled, 1 oz. 11.4
Breadnut tree seeds, dried, 1 oz. 22.5
Broad beans, fresh, boiled, drained, 4 oz. 11.5
Broad beans, mature, boiled, ½ cup 16.7
Broad beans, canned, with liquid, ½ cup 15.9
Broccoli, fresh:
    raw, 8.7-oz. stalk 7.9
    boiled, drained, 1 stalk, 6.3 oz. 9.1
    boiled, drained, chopped, ½ cup 3.9
Broccoli, frozen, boiled, drained, 1 cup 9.8
Broccoli rabe, fresh, cooked, ½ cup 3.0
Brownie, 2-oz. piece 35.8
Brownie mix, prepared, 2"-square piece 20.4
Brussels sprouts, fresh:
    boiled, .7-oz. piece 1.8
    boiled, drained, ½ cup 6.8
Brussels sprouts, frozen, boiled, drained, ½ cup 6.5
Buckwheat, grain, ¼ cup 30.4
Buckwheat flour, ¼ cup 21.2
Buckwheat groats, roasted, cooked, 1 cup 39.5
Bulgur, cooked, 1 cup 33.8
Bun, sweet, refrigerated, cinnamon, iced, 1 piece .. 45.0
Burbot, without added ingredients 0
Burdock root, boiled, 1" pieces, ½ cup 13.2
Butter, regular, 1 stick or 4 oz. 0
Butter beans, see "Lima beans"
Butterbur, fresh, boiled, drained, 4 oz. 2.4
Butterbur, canned, chopped, ½ cup 2
Butterfish, without added ingredients 0
Buttermilk, see "Milk"
Butternut, dried, shelled, 1 oz. 3.4
Butternut squash, baked, cubed, ½ cup 10.7
Butterscotch topping, 2 tbsp. 30.0

Cabbage, fresh:
    raw, shredded, ½ cup 1.9
    boiled, drained, shredded, ½ cup 3.4
Cabbage, Chinese, fresh:
    bok choy, raw, shredded, ½ cup 8
    bok choy, boiled, drained, shredded, ½ cup 1.5
    pe-tsai, raw, shredded, ½ cup 1.2
Cabbage, red, fresh:
    raw, shredded, ½ cup 2.1
    boiled, drained, shredded, ½ cup 3.5
Cabbage, savoy, boiled, drained, shredded, ½ cup 4.0
Cactus pads, fresh:
    raw, sliced, 1 cup 2.9
    cooked, 1 cup 4.9
Cactus pads, canned, 2 tbsp. 1.0
Cake:
    angel food, ¹⁄₁₂ of 12-oz. cake 16.4
    Boston cream, ⅙ of 19.5-oz. cake 39.5
    cheesecake, 2-oz. piece 14.4
    chocolate, chocolate icing, ⅛ of 18-oz. cake 34.9
    coffee cake, cheese, 2-oz. piece 25.3
    coffee cake, cinnamon crumb, 2-oz. piece 26.4
    fruitcake, 2-oz. piece 35.3
    pound cake, 2-oz. piece 29.8
    sponge cake, ¹⁄₁₂ of 16-oz. cake 23.2
    yellow, chocolate icing, ⅛ of 18-oz. cake 35.5
Cake, mix, prepared, ¹⁄₁₂ of 9" cake, except as noted:
    angel food 29.3
    carrot, with icing 32.7
    cheesecake, no-bake, ⅛ of 9" cake 35.2
    chocolate, devil's food, or fudge, without icing .. 31.8
    chocolate, German, coconut icing 55.1
    white or yellow, without icing 34.4
Cake, snack, crème-filled:
    chocolate icing, 1.8-oz. piece 30.1
    sponge, 1.5-oz. piece 27.1
Candy:
    (*Almond Joy*), 1.6-oz. bar 27.0
    almonds, chocolate coated, 1.4 oz. 20.0
    (*Baby Ruth*), 2.1-oz. bar 37.0
    bridge mix (*Brach's*), 16 pieces, 1.4 oz. 26.0
    (*Butterfinger*), 2.1-oz. bar 43.0
    candy corn (*Brach's*), 26 pieces, 1.4 oz. 35.0
    caramels, 1 oz. 21.8
    chocolate, dark or sweet, 1 oz. 16.9
    chocolate, milk, 1 oz. 16.8

(*5th Avenue*), 2-oz. bar 35.0
gum, chewing, 1 piece 2.9
hard, 1 oz. 27.8
hard, fruit or mint (*LifeSavers*), 2 pieces 5.0
jelly beans, 10 large or 1 oz. 26.4
licorice, candy coated (*Good & Plenty*),
    1.75 oz. 43.0
licorice twists (*Twizzlers*), 4 pieces, 1.6 oz. 34.0
(*M&M's* Plain), 1 oz. 19.3
malt balls, chocolate coated, 1.4 oz. 30.0
marshmallows (*Kraft Jet-Puffed*), 1 oz. 23.0
(*Milk Duds*), 13 pieces, 1.4 oz. 28.0
(*Milky Way*), 2-oz. bar 41.0
mint, chocolate coated (*Junior Mints*), 1.4 oz. .. 30.0
(*Mounds*), 1.7-oz. bar 29.0
(*Mr. Goodbar*), 1.7-oz. bar 27.0
nonpareils (*Sno•Caps*), ¼ cup, 1.4 oz. 30.0
(*PayDay*), 1.8-oz. bar 28.0
peanut bar (*Planters*), 1.6 oz. 22.0
peanuts, chocolate coated, 1 oz. 14.0
peanuts, French burnt (*Brach's*), 1.4 oz. 29.0
peppermint, chocolate coated (*York*), 1.4 oz. 32.0
raisins, chocolate coated (*Raisinets*), ¼ cup,
    1.4 oz. 32.0
(*Reese's Peanut Butter Cups*), 1.5 oz. 23.0
(*Reese's Pieces*), 1.5 oz. 26.0
(*Rolo*), 1.7-oz. package 31.0
(*Snickers*) 2.1-oz. bar 35.0
spearmint leaves (*Brach's*), 5 pieces, 1.4 oz. 34.0
spice drops (*Brach's*), 12 pieces, 1.4 oz. 33.0
strawberry twists (*Twizzlers*), 4 pieces, 1.6 oz. .. 36.0
(*3 Musketeers*), 2.13-oz. bar 46.0
toffee bar, 1.4 oz. 24.0
truffles, assorted, 1.5 oz. 27.0
Cane syrup, 1 tbsp. 13.4
Cantaloupe:
½ of 5" melon 22.3
cubed, 1 cup 13.4
Capers, 1 tbsp. 1.0
Capon, without added ingredients 0
Carambola, fresh, 1 medium, 4.7 oz. 9.9
Caramel syrup, 2 tbsp. 25.0
Caraway seeds, 1 tsp. 1.1
Cardamom, ground, 1 tsp. 1.4
Carissa, 1 medium, .8 oz. 2.7
Carp, without added ingredients 0
Carrot, fresh:
raw, whole, 7½" long, 2.8 oz. 7.3
raw, shredded, ½ cup 5.6

raw, baby, medium, 2¾" long 8
boiled, drained, sliced, ½ cup 8.2
Carrot, canned, sliced, drained, ½ cup 4.0
Carrot, frozen, sliced, boiled, drained, ½ cup 6.0
Casaba melon, ⅒ of 7¾" melon, or 1 cup 10.2
Cashews:
dry-roasted, 18 medium, 1 oz. 9.3
oil-roasted, 18 medium, 1 oz. 8.1
Catfish, without added ingredients 0
Cauliflower, fresh:
raw, 3 florets, 5 oz. 2.9
raw or boiled, drained, 1" pieces, ½ cup 2.6
green, boiled, drained, 1" pieces, ½ cup 3.9
Cauliflower, frozen, boiled, drained, ½ cup 3.4
Caviar (see also "Roe"), black or red, 1 tbsp. 6
Celery:
raw, 7½"-stalk, 1.6 oz. 1.5
raw, diced, ½ cup 2.2
boiled, drained, diced, ½ cup 3.0
Celery, dried, flakes or seeds, 1 tsp. 9
Cereal, ready-to-eat:
bran flakes, 1 cup 22.0
bran flakes, with raisins, 1 cup 43.0
cornflakes, 1 cup 26.0
granola, ½ cup 37.0
kamut or spelt flakes, 1 cup 25.0
multigrain, 1 cup 28.0
oats or oat bran flakes, 1 cup 24.0
rice, crisps, 1 cup 25.0
rice, puffed, 1 cup 15.0
wheat, 1 cup 24.0
wheat, shredded, 2 pieces or 1 cup 38.0
Cereal, cooking/hot, uncooked:
multigrain, ¼ cup 28.0
oatmeal, oats, or rolled oats, ½ cup 27.0
wheat, farina, 3 tbsp. 26.0
Chayote, raw, 1 medium, 7.2 oz. 11.0
Cheese, 1 oz., except as noted:
American, processed 5
asiago 2
blue or bleu 7
brick 8
Brie, Camembert, or Gruyère 1
caraway 9
cheddar 4
Cheshire 1.4
Colby 7
cottage, creamed, 4% fat, large curd, ½ cup 2.8
cottage, creamed, 4% fat, with fruit, ½ cup 5.2

cottage, 2% fat, ½ cup 4.1
cottage, 1% fat, ½ cup 3.1
cream cheese, 2 tbsp. or 1 oz. 8
Edam or Fontina 4
feta 1.2
Gjetost 12.1
goat, semisoft type 7
goat, soft type 3
Gouda 6
Limburger 1
Monterey Jack 2
mozzarella, part skim 8
mozzarella, whole milk 6
Muenster 3
Parmesan 1.1
Parmesan, grated, 1 tbsp. 2
Port du Salut 2
provolone 6
ricotta, part skim, ½ cup 6.3
ricotta, whole milk, ½ cup 3.7
Romano 1.0
Roquefort 6
Swiss, natural 1.0
Swiss, processed 6
Cheese dip or sauce, 2 tbsp. 2.0
Cheese spread, American, processed, 1 oz. 2.5
Cherimoya, trimmed, 1 oz. 6.8
Cherry, fresh:
    sour, red, ½ cup, with pits 6.3
    sour, red, ½ cup, red, pitted 9.4
    sweet, with pits, ½ cup 12.0
    sweet, 10 medium 11.3
Cherry, canned, ½ cup:
    sour, pitted, in light syrup 24.3
    sour, pitted, in heavy syrup 29.8
    sweet, in light syrup 21.8
    sweet, in heavy syrup 27.4
Cherry juice blend, 8 fl. oz. 30.0
Chervil, dried, 1 tsp. 3
Chestnut, Chinese, shelled, dried, 1 oz. 22.7
Chestnut, European:
    roasted, peeled, 1 oz. 15.0
    roasted, peeled, 1 cup, 17 kernels 75.7
Chicken, meat only, without added ingredients 0
Chicken giblets, simmered, chopped, 1 cup 1.4
Chicken gravy, can or jar, ¼ cup 3.5
Chicken lunch meat, breast, oven-roasted, 2 oz. 2.0
Chickpeas, see "Garbanzo beans"
Chicory, witloof, 5-7" head, 1.9 oz. 2.1

Chicory greens, chopped, ½ cup 4.2
Chicory root, 1" piece, ½ cup 7.9
Chili, canned:
    with beans, 1 cup 30.0
    without beans, 1 cup 17.0
Chili pepper, see "Pepper, chili"
Chili powder, 1 tbsp. 4.1
Chili sauce, tomato, 1 tbsp. 5.0
Chitterlings, pork 0
Chives, fresh, chopped, 1 tbsp. 1
Chocolate, see "Candy"
Chocolate, baking:
    bar, unsweetened, .5 oz. 8.0
    chips or morsels, .5 oz. or 1 tbsp. 10.0
    semisweet, .5 oz. 9.0
Chocolate milk, 1 cup 25.9
Chocolate syrup, 2 tbsp. 25.0
Chocolate topping, hot fudge, 2 tbsp. 23.0
Chorizo, pork and beef, 2-oz. link 1.0
Chutney, mango, Major Grey's, 1 tbsp. 12.0
Cilantro, see "Coriander"
Cinnamon, ground, 1 tsp. 2.1
Cisco, without added ingredients 0
Clam, meat only:
    raw, 9 large or 20 small, 6.3 oz. 4.6
    boiled, poached, or steamed, 4 oz. 5.8
Clam, canned, drained, 2 oz. or ¼ cup 2.1
Clam chowder, see "Soup"
Clam dip, 2 tbsp. 2.0
Clam juice, 1 cup 1.0
Clam sauce, canned, ½ cup 8.0
Cloves, ground, 1 tsp. 1.3
Cocktail sauce, see "Seafood sauce"
Cocoa, Dutch or unsweetened, 1 tbsp. 3.0
Cocoa mix, 1-oz. pkt. 22.5
Coconut, fresh, 1 piece, 2" x 2" x ½", 1.6 oz. 6.9
Coconut, dried, flaked, sweetened, 2 tbsp. 6.0
Coconut milk, canned, 2 tbsp. 1.0
Cod, without added ingredients 0
Coffee, brewed, 6 fl. oz. 8
Cold cuts, see specific listings
Coleslaw, refrigerated, ¼ cup 19.0
Collard greens, fresh:
    raw, chopped, ½ cup 1.3
    boiled, drained, chopped, ½ cup 3.9
Collard greens, frozen, boiled, drained, ½ cup 6.1
Conch, baked or broiled, 4 oz. 1.9
Cookie, 1 oz., except as noted:
    animal crackers 21.0

butter 19.5
chocolate chip 18.9
chocolate sandwich, crème-filled 19.9
chocolate wafer 20.5
fudge, cake-type 22.2
ginger snaps 21.8
graham cracker, plain or honey 21.8
graham cracker, chocolate coated 18.8
ladyfinger 16.9
oatmeal, fat free 22.2
peanut butter 16.7
peanut butter sandwich 18.6
raisin, soft type 19.3
shortbread, pecan 16.5
sugar 19.2
vanilla sandwich, crème-filled 20.4
vanilla wafer 20.2
Cookie mix, refrigerated dough, baked:
chocolate chip, 1 oz. 19.3
oatmeal or sugar, 1 oz. 18.6
peanut butter, 1 oz. 16.2
Coriander, fresh, ¼ cup 1
Coriander, dried:
leaf, 1 tsp. 3
seeds, 1 tsp. 1.0
Corn, fresh:
baby, .28-oz. ear 2.0
golden or white, raw, 5-oz. ear 27.2
golden or white, kernels, boiled, drained, ½ cup .. 20.6
white, boiled, drained, 2.72-oz. ear 19.3
Corn, canned:
kernels, drained, ½ cup 15.2
cream style, ½ cup 23.2
Corn, frozen, kernels, ½ cup 18.3
Corn, whole-grain, ¼ cup 30.8
Corn chips/crisps, 1 oz.:
cheese flavor, twists or puffs 15.3
tortilla, low fat 22.7
tortilla, nacho flavor 17.7
Cornflake crumbs (*Kellogg's*), 2 tbsp. 9.0
Corn flour:
whole grain, ¼ cup 22.5
masa, ¼ cup 21.8
Corn grits, cooked, ½ cup 15.7
Corn syrup, dark or light, 2 tbsp. 31.0
Cornish hen, without added ingredients 0
Cornmeal (see also "Corn flour" and "Polenta"):
self-rising, dry, ¼ cup 21.4
whole-grain, dry, ¼ cup 23.5

Cornstarch, 1 tbsp. 7.0
Couscous, cooked, ½ cup 20.8
Cowpeas (see also "Black-eyed peas"), boiled,
    drained:
    immature seeds, ½ cup 16.8
    leafy tips, chopped, ½ cup 7
    pods, with seeds, ½ cup 3.3
Crab, meat only, boiled or steamed:
    Alaska king, blue, or queen, 4 oz. 0
    Dungeness, 4 oz. 1.1
Crab, canned, 4 oz. 0
"Crab," imitation, from surimi, 1 oz. 3.0
Crab apple, fresh, sliced, ½ cup 11.0
Cracker, 1 oz.:
    cheese 16.5
    cheese sandwich, peanut butter filled 16.2
    crispbread, rye 23.2
    matzo, plain 23.8
    rye wafers 22.8
    saltines 20.4
    saltines, fat free, low sodium 24.0
    sandwich, cheese filled 17.4
    sandwich, peanut butter filled 16.6
    soda or water 22.0
    soup or oyster 21.0
    wheat 18.5
    whole wheat 19.4
Cracker meal, ¼ cup 23.3
Cranberry, fresh, raw, whole ½ cup 6.0
Cranberry, dried, ⅓ cup, 1.4 oz. 33.0
Cranberry beans, boiled, ½ cup 21.5
Cranberry juice cocktail, 8 fl. oz. 34.0
Cranberry sauce, whole or jellied, ¼ cup 26.0
Crayfish, without added ingredients 0
Cream, 1 tbsp.:
    half-and-half, light, coffee or table 6
    medium (25% fat), 1 tbsp. 5
    whipping, 1 tbsp. (2 tbsp. whipped) 4
Cream, sour, 2 tbsp.:
    regular 1.0
    light or nondairy 2.0
    nonfat 4.0
Cream topping, 2 tbsp. 2.0
Creamer, nondairy, powder, 1 tsp. 1.1
Creamer, nondairy:
Crème fraîche, 2 tbsp. .... <1.0
Cress, garden:
    raw, ½ cup 1.4
    boiled, drained, ½ cup 2.6

Croaker, Atlantic, without added ingredients 0
Croissant:
  butter, 1-oz. piece 13.0
  cheese, 1.5-oz. piece 19.7
Crookneck squash, sliced, boiled, drained, ½ cup 3.9
Crookneck squash, canned, cut, drained, ½ cup 3.2
Crookneck squash, frozen, boiled, sliced, ½ cup 5.3
Croutons, plain, ½ cup 11.0
Cucumber, with peel:
  1 medium, 8¼" long 8.3
  sliced, ½ cup 1.4
Cumin seeds, ground, 1 tsp. 9
Currants:
  fresh, black, European, ½ cup 8.6
  fresh, red or white, ½ cup 7.7
  dried, Zante, ½ cup 53.3
Curry powder, 1 tsp. 1.2
Cusk, without added ingredients 0
Custard, mix, prepared with milk:
  egg, ½ cup 23.4
  flan or caramel, ½ cup 25.4
Custard apple, trimmed, 1 oz. 7.1
Cuttlefish, meat only, boiled or steamed, 4 oz. 1.9

D–E

Daikon, see "Radish, Oriental"
Dandelion greens, boiled, drained, chopped, ½ cup .. 3.3
Danish pastry, 1 piece:
  cheese, 4¼" diam., 2.5 oz. 26.4
  cinnamon, 4¼" diam., 2.3 oz. 29.0
  fruit, 4¼" diam., 2.5 oz. 34.0
  nut, 4¼" diam., 2.3 oz. 29.7
Date, domestic, dried:
  10 pieces, 2.9 oz. 61.0
  pitted, ½ cup 65.4
Dill seeds, 1 tsp. 1.2
Dill weed, fresh, 1 cup 6
Dill weed, dried, 1 tsp. 6
Dock, boiled, drained, 4 oz. 3.3
Dolphin fish, without added ingredients 0
Donut, 1 piece:
  cake type, chocolate frosted, 1.5 oz. 20.6
  cake type, chocolate, sugared or glazed, 1.5 oz. .. 24.1
  cake type, wheat, sugared or glazed, 1.6 oz. 19.2
  crueller, glazed, 1.4 oz. 24.4
  yeast type, glazed, 2.1 oz. 26.6
  yeast type, jelly filled, 3 oz. 33.2

Drum, freshwater, without added ingredients 0
Duck, meat only, without added ingredients 0
Eel, without added ingredients 0
Egg, chicken:
    raw, whole, 1 large 6
    raw, white or yolk, 1 large 3
    cooked, boiled, poached, or scrambled, 1 large 6
    cooked, hard-boiled, chopped, 1 cup 1.5
Egg, substitute, ¼ cup 1.0
Egg roll wrapper, 7"-square piece 18.5
Eggnog, nonalcoholic, ½ cup 17.2
Eggplant, fresh:
    raw, 1" pieces, ½ cup 2.5
    boiled, drained, 1" cubes, ½ cup 3.2
Elderberries, ½ cup 13.3
Endive or escarole, chopped, ½ cup 8
Endive, Belgian, see "Chicory, witloof"
Eppaw, raw, ½ cup 15.8

F

Farina, whole-grain, cooked, 1 cup 24.6
Farro, see "Spelt"
Fava beans, see "Broad beans"
Feijoa, raw:
    with skin, 1 medium, 2.3 oz. 5.3
    pureed, ½ cup 12.9
Fennel, bulb, fresh, raw:
    8.3-oz. bulb 17.1
    sliced, 1 cup 6.3
Fennel seeds, 1 tsp. 1.1
Fenugreek seeds, 1 tsp. 2.2
Fiddlehead fern, fresh, 4 oz. 6.3
Fig, fresh:
    1 large, 2.3 oz. 12.3
    1 medium, 1.8 oz. 9.6
Fig, canned:
    in light syrup, ½ cup 22.6
    in heavy syrup, ½ cup 29.7
Fig, dried, 5 figs, 3.3 oz. 61.0
Filberts, see "Hazelnuts"
Fillo dough, frozen, sheets, 2 oz. 37.0
Fish, see specific listings
Fish, frozen, breaded:
    fillet, heated, 2-oz. piece 13.5
    sticks, heated, 1-oz. piece 6.7
Fish oil, all varieties, 2 tbsp. 0
Flatfish or flounder, without added ingredients 0

Flax seeds, 3 tbsp. 10.0
Flour, see "Wheat flour" and specific listings
Frankfurter, 1 link:
    beef, 5" link, 2 oz. 1.0
    beef and pork, 5" link, 2 oz. 1.5
    cheese, 1.5-oz. link 6
French toast, frozen, 2.1-oz. piece 19.0
Frosting, ready-to-spread, chocolate, 2 tbsp. 22.0
Fruit or fruit juice, see specific listings
Fruit, mixed, canned:
    in juice, ½ cup 14.7
    in light syrup, ½ cup 18.8
    in heavy syrup, ½ cup 24.2
Fruit, mixed, candied, 1 oz. 23.4
Fruit, mixed, dried, ¼ cup, 1.4 oz. 28.0
Fruit bar, frozen, 1 bar 15.6
Fruit punch drink, 8 fl. oz. 29.0
Fruit snack/leather, all fruits, ¾-oz. roll 17.7
Fruit spread, all fruits, 1 tbsp. 10.0

G
carbohydrates

Garbanzo beans, boiled, ½ cup 22.5
Garbanzo beans, canned, with liquid,
  ½ cup 27.1
Garlic, fresh:
    1 clove, .1 oz. 1.0
    minced, 1 tsp. 2.9
Garlic pepper, 1 tsp. 1.8
Garlic powder, 1 tsp. 2.3
Garlic salt, 1 tsp. 5
Gelatin, unflavored, 1 pkt. 0
Gelatin dessert mix, prepared, ½ cup 17.0
Ginger, trimmed root, sliced, ¼ cup 3.6
Ginger, ground, 1 tsp. 1.3
Ginger, pickled, Japanese, 1 oz. 2.1
Ginkgo nut, shelled, canned, drained, 1 oz. 6.3
Goose, meat only, without added ingredients 0
Gooseberries, fresh, ½ cup 7.6
Granola, see "Cereal, ready-to-eat"
Granola bar, 1 oz.:
    hard, plain 18.3
    hard, chocolate chip 20.4
    hard, peanut butter 17.7
    soft, plain 19.1
    soft, chocolate chip 19.6
    soft, chocolate chip, chocolate coated 18.1
    soft, nut and raisin 16.0

soft, peanut butter 18.2
soft, peanut butter, chocolate coated 15.1
soft, raisin 18.8
Grape, fresh:
American type (slip-skin), 10 medium 4.1
American type, peeled and seeded, ½ cup 7.9
European type (adherent skin), seedless,
10 medium 8.9
European type, seedless or seeded, ½ cup 14.2
Grape drink, 8 fl. oz. 28.8
Grape juice, 8 fl. oz. 37.7
Grapefruit, fresh, all areas:
½ large, 4.7 oz. 13.4
sections, 1 cup 18.6
pink or red, ½ medium, 3¾" 9.5
pink, red, or white, sections, 1 cup 17.7
white, ½ medium, 3¾" 9.9
Grapefruit, canned:
in juice, with liquid, ½ cup 11.4
in light syrup, with liquid, ½ cup 19.6
Grapefruit juice, 8 fl. oz.:
fresh, pink or white 22.7
canned, unsweetened 22.1
frozen*, unsweetened 24.0
Gravy, see specific listings
Great northern beans, dry, boiled, ½ cup 18.6
Great northern beans, canned, with liquid,
½ cup 27.6
Green beans, fresh:
raw, ½ cup 3.9
boiled, drained, ½ cup 4.9
Green beans, canned, cuts, with liquid, ½ cup 4.2
Green beans, frozen, boiled, drained, ½ cup 4.4
Green peas, see "Peas, green"
Grits, see "Corn grits"
Grouper, without added ingredients 0
Guacamole, refrigerated, 2 tbsp. 2.5
Guava:
½ cup 9.8
strawberry, ½ cup 21.2
Guava sauce, ½ cup 11.3
Guinea hen, meat only, without added ingredients 0

H   carbohydrates

Haddock, fresh or smoked, without added
ingredients 0
Halibut, Atlantic/Pacific, without added ingredients .. 0

Halvah, 2 oz. 18.0
Ham, fresh, without added ingredients 0
Ham, cured, meat only:
    whole leg, unheated, 4 oz. or 1 cup 1
    whole leg, roasted, 4 oz. or 1 cup diced 0
    boneless, 11% fat, unheated, 4 oz. 3.5
    boneless, extra lean, 5% fat, unheated, 4 oz. 1.1
    boneless, extra lean, 5% fat, roasted, 4 oz. 1.7
Ham, refrigerated or canned, roasted, 4 oz. 6
Ham lunch meat, baked or smoked, 2 oz. 2.0
Ham patty, grilled, 4 oz. 1.9
Hazelnut, shelled:
    dry-roasted, salted, 1 oz. 5.1
    oil-roasted, salted, 1 oz. 5.4
Head cheese, pork, 2 oz. 0
Heart, braised or simmered, beef or pork, 4 oz. 5
Herbs, see specific listings
Herring, fresh or cured, without added ingredients 0
Herring, canned, see "Sardine"
Herring, pickled, in jars:, 4 oz. 10.9
Hickory nut, dried, shelled, 1 oz. 5.2
Hoisin sauce, 1 tbsp. 7.1
Hollandaise sauce, in jars, 2 tbsp. 1.0
Hominy, dry, white (*Goya*), ¼ cup 39.0
Hominy, canned, ¼ cup 11.4
Honey, 1 tbsp. 17.0
Honey roll sausage, beef, 1 oz. 6
Honeydew melon:
    ¹⁄₁₀ melon, 7" x 2" 11.8
    cubed, 1 cup 15.6
Horseradish, prepared, 1 tbsp. 1.0
Horseradish sauce, 1 tsp. 1.0
Hot dog, see "Frankfurter"
Hot sauce, 1 tsp. 0
Hubbard squash:
    baked, cubed, ½ cup 11.0
    boiled, drained, mashed, ½ cup 7.6
Hummus, 2 tbsp. 4.2
Hyacinth beans, dried, boiled, ½ cup 20.1

I–J–K
carbohydrates

Ice, ½ cup:
    lime, ½ cup 31.3
    pineapple-coconut, ½ cup 23.0
Ice bar, fruit flavor, reduced calorie, 1 bar 3.2
Ice cream, ½ cup:
    chocolate 18.6

chocolate, rich 25.7
strawberry 18.2
vanilla 15.5
vanilla, rich 23.7
vanilla, soft-serve 19.0
"Ice cream," nondairy, chocolate, ½ cup 24.0
Ice-cream cone, unfilled, sugar or waffle, 1 piece .. 10.0
Icing, cake, see "Frosting"
Jackfruit, fresh, trimmed, 1 oz. 6.8
Jackfruit, canned, in syrup, ½ cup 21.3
Jalapeño, see "Pepper, jalapeño"
Jam/preserves (see also "Fruit spread"), fruit,
1 tbsp. 12.9
Java plum, 3 medium, .4 oz. 1.4
Jelly, fruit, 1 tbsp. 13.5
Jerusalem artichoke, sliced, ½ cup 13.1
Jicama, see "Yam beans"
Jujube, dried, 1 oz. 20.1
Jute, potherb, boiled, drained, ½ cup 3.1
Kale, fresh, boiled, drained, chopped, ½ cup 3.7
Kale, frozen, boiled, drained, chopped, ½ cup 3.4
Kale, Chinese, fresh, cooked, 1 cup 3.3
Kale, Scotch, boiled, drained, chopped, ½ cup 3.7
Ketchup, 1 tbsp. 4.0
Kidney beans, dry, boiled, ½ cup 20.1
Kidney beans, canned, with liquid, ½ cup 20.0
Kidney beans, sprouted, raw, ½ cup 3.8
Kidneys, braised:
beef or lamb, 4 oz. 1.1
pork or veal, 4 oz. or 1 cup chopped 0
Kielbasa, 2 oz. 2.0
Kiwi, fresh:
1 large, 3.7 oz. 13.5
1 medium, 3.1 oz. 11.3
Knockwurst, pork and beef, 2-oz. link 2.0
Kohlrabi, boiled, drained, sliced, ½ cup 5.5
Kumquat, 1 medium, .7 oz. 3.1

L

carbohydrates

Lamb, meat only, without added ingredients 0
Lamb's quarters, boiled, drained, chopped,
½ cup 4.5
Lard, pork, 1 tbsp. 0
Leek, fresh, with lower leaf portion:
raw, chopped, ½ cup 7.4
boiled, drained, 4.4-oz. leek 9.5
boiled, drained, chopped, ½ cup 4.0

Leek, freeze-dried, 1 tbsp. 2
Lemon, fresh:
    2⅛" lemon, 3.8 oz. 11.6
    peeled, 2⅛" lemon 5.4
Lemon curd, 1 tbsp. 13.0
Lemon grass, fresh, ½ cup 8.5
Lemon juice, fresh, 1 tbsp. 1.3
Lemon peel, fresh, 1 tbsp. 1.0
Lemon pepper, 1 tsp. 1.5
Lemonade, pink or white, 8 fl. oz. 26.0
Lentil, cooked, ½ cup 19.9
Lentil, sprouted, raw, ½ cup 8.4
Lettuce:
    bibb or Boston, 1 head, 5" diam. 3.8
    bibb or Boston, 2 inner leaves 4
    iceberg, 1 head, 6" diam. 11.3
    iceberg, shredded, 1 cup 1.2
    leaf/looseleaf, shredded, ½ cup 1.0
    romaine or cos, shredded, ½ cup 7
    romaine hearts, 6 leaves, 3 oz. 3.0
Lima beans:
    immature, ½ cup, boiled, drained 20.1
    mature, dry, baby, boiled, ½ cup 21.2
    mature, boiled, ½ cup 19.6
Lima beans, canned, with liquid, ½ cup 17.2
Lima beans, frozen, boiled, drained, ½ cup 16.0
Lime, fresh, 2"-diam. lime 7.1
Lime juice, fresh, 1 tbsp. 1.4
Limeade, frozen. diluted, 8 fl. oz. 27.1
Ling or Ling cod, without added ingredients 0
Liquor, pure distilled (gin, scotch, vodka, etc.),
    1 fl. oz. 0
Liver:
    beef, pan-fried, 4 oz. 8.9
    calves (veal), braised, 4 oz. 4.3
    calves (veal), pan-fried, 4 oz. 5.1
    chicken, simmered, chopped, 1 cup 1.2
    chicken, pan-fried, 4 oz. 1.3
    goose, raw, 1 oz. 1.8
    lamb, pan-fried, 4 oz. 4.3
    pork, braised, 4 oz. 4.3
    turkey, simmered, 4 oz. 3.9
    turkey, simmered, chopped, 1 cup 4.8
Liver cheese, pork, 2 oz. 1.8
Liverwurst, 2 oz. 1.2
Liverwurst spread, ¼ cup, 2 oz. 3.2
Lobster, northern, meat only:
    boiled or steamed, 4 oz. 1.5
    boiled or steamed, 1 cup, 5.1 oz. 1.9

Lobster, spiny, see "Spiny lobster"
Loganberries, fresh, 1 cup 21.5
Loganberries, frozen, ½ cup 9.6
Long beans, see "Yard-long beans"
Longan, fresh, seeded, 1 oz. 4.3
Longan, dried, 1 oz. 21.0
Loquat, 1 large, .7 oz. 2.4
Lotus root, boiled, drained, ½ cup 9.6
Lotus seeds, dried, 1 oz. 18.3
Lunch meat, see specific listings
Lunch meat, canned, 2 oz. 1.0
Lupin, boiled, ½ cup 8.2
Lychee, fresh:
   1 fruit, .3 oz. 1.6
   shelled, 1 cup 31.4
Lychee, dried, 10 fruits, .7 oz. 17.7

                                 carbohydrates

Macadamia nut, shelled:
   raw or dried, whole or halves, ¼ cup 4.6
   dry-roasted or oil-roasted, 1 oz. 3.8
Macaroni (see also "Pasta"), cooked:
   enriched, elbows, 1 cup 39.7
   enriched, spirals, 1 cup 38.0
   small shells, 1 cup 32.6
   vegetable, enriched, spirals, 1 cup 35.7
   whole-wheat, elbows, 1 cup 37.2
Macaroni and cheese, canned, 1 cup 32.0
Mace, ground, 1 tsp. 9
Mackerel, without added ingredients 0
Mahi mahi, without added ingredients 0
Malanga, fresh, sliced, ½ cup 16.0
Malted milk powder, natural, 3 tbsp. 15.0
Mammy apple, ½ of 25-oz. fruit 52.9
Mango, fresh:
   10.6-oz. fruit, 7.3 oz. trimmed 35.2
   sliced, 1 cup 28.1
Mango, frozen, chunks, 1 cup 21.0
Mangosteen, canned, in syrup, ½ cup 6.7
Maple syrup, pure, ¼ cup 53.0
Margarine, regular, all varieties, ¼ cup 0
Marjoram, dried, 1 tsp. 4
Marmalade, orange, 1 tbsp. 13.3
Marrow squash, raw, trimmed, 1 oz. 1.0
Marshmallow topping, 2 tbsp. 22.5
Mayonnaise:
   real, 1 tbsp. 4

reduced fat or light, 1 tbsp. 1.5
Mayonnaise dressing, 1 tbsp. 2.0
Meat, potted, ¼ cup 0
Meat tenderizer, 1 tsp. 1.2
Melon, see specific melon listings
Melon balls, frozen, cantaloupe/honeydew, ½ cup 6.9
Milk, 8 fl. oz.:
    buttermilk, cultured 11.7
    whole, 3.3% fat 11.4
    reduced or low fat, 2% or 1% 11.7
    reduced or low fat, 2% or 1%, protein fortified .. 13.5
    skim or fat free 11.9
Milk, canned, 2 tbsp.:
    condensed, sweetened 21.0
    evaporated, whole 3.2
    evaporated, skim 3.9
Milk, chocolate, see "Chocolate milk"
Milk, dry:
    buttermilk, sweet cream, 1 tbsp. 3.2
    whole, 1 oz. 10.9
    nonfat, regular, ¼ cup 15.6
    instant, 3.2-oz. pkt. 35.5
Milk, goat, 8 fl. oz. 11.0
"Milk," nondairy (see also "Soy milk"), 1 cup 15.0
Milkfish, without added ingredients 0
Millet, cooked, ½ cup 28.4
Mint, fresh, spearmint, 2 tbsp. 9
Mint, dried, spearmint, 1 tbsp. 8
Miso, soy paste, ½ cup 38.6
Molasses, dark or light, 1 tbsp. 13.8
Monkfish, without added ingredients 0
Mortadella, beef and pork, 2 oz. 1.7
Mother's loaf, pork, 2 oz. 4.1
Muffin, 2-oz. piece:
    blueberry 27.4
    corn 29.0
    English, plain 28.2
    English, wheat 25.5
    oat bran 27.5
Muffin mix, prepared, 1.75-oz. piece:
    blueberry 24.4
    corn 24.8
    wheat bran 23.3
Mulberries, fresh, ½ cup 6.9
Mullet, without added ingredients 0
Mung beans, dry, boiled, ½ cup 19.3
Mung bean sprouts, raw, 1 cup 6.2
Mung bean sprouts, canned, drained, 1 cup 2.7
Mungo beans, boiled, ½ cup 16.5

Mushroom, fresh:
    common, raw, pieces or slices, ½ cup 1.5
    common, boiled, drained, pieces, ½ cup 4.0
    crimini, raw, brown or Italian, .5-oz. piece 6
    enoki, raw, 1 large, 4½" long 4
    oyster, raw, 1 small, .5 oz. 9
    portobello, raw, 1 oz. 1.4
    shiitake, cooked, 4 medium or ½ cup pieces 10.4
Mushroom, canned, drained:
    common, whole or sliced, drained, ½ cup 3.9
    straw, ½ cup 4.2
Mushroom, dried:
    cloud ear, .2-oz. piece 3.3
    porcini, ⅓ oz., 5 pieces 2.0
    shiitake, 4 medium, .5 oz. 11.3
Mushroom gravy, canned, ¼ cup 3.0
Mussels, blue, meat only, boiled or steamed,
    4 oz. 8.4
Mussels, smoked, canned, ¼ cup 3.0
Mustard, prepared, 1 tsp. .... <1.0
Mustard greens, fresh:
    raw, chopped, 1 oz. or ½ cup 1.4
    boiled, drained, ½ cup 1.5
Mustard greens, canned, ½ cup 4.0
Mustard greens, frozen, boiled, drained, 1 cup 4.7
Mustard powder, 1 tsp. 3
Mustard seeds, 1 tsp. 1.2
Mustard spinach, boiled, drained, chopped, 1 cup .. 5.0

 carbohydrates

Natto, ½ cup 12.6
Navy beans, boiled, ½ cup 24.0
Navy beans, canned, with liquid, ½ cup 26.8
Navy beans, sprouted, ½ cup 6.8
Nectarine:
    1 medium, 2½" diam. 16.0
    sliced, ½ cup 8.1
Noodle, Asian:
    cellophane or long rice, dry, 2 oz. 48.8
    chow mein, dry, ½ cup 13.0
    rice, dry, 2 oz. 47.0
    soba, cooked, 1 cup 24.4
    somen, cooked, 1 cup 48.5
    udon, cooked, 4 oz. 23.0
Noodle, egg:
    cooked, 1 cup 39.7
    cooked, spinach, 1 cup 38.8

Nopales/Nopalitos, see "Cactus pads"
Nutmeg, ground, 1 tsp. 1.1
Nuts, see specific listings
Nuts, mixed, 1 oz.:
    dry-roasted, with peanuts 7.2
    oil-roasted, with peanuts 6.1
    oil-roasted, without peanuts 6.3
Oat (see also "Cereal"):
    whole-grain, dry, ¼ cup 25.8
    rolled or oatmeal, dry, ¼ cup 13.5
    rolled or oatmeal, cooked, ½ cup 12.6
Oat bran:
    dry, ¼ cup 15.6
    cooked, ½ cup 12.5
Ocean perch, without added ingredients 0
Octopus, meat only, boiled or steamed,
    4 oz. 5.0
Octopus, canned, 2 oz. 3.0
Oheloberry, ½ cup 4.8
Oil, all varieties 0
Okra, fresh:
    raw, sliced, ½ cup 3.8
    boiled, drained, 8 pods, 3" x ⅝" 6.1
    boiled, drained, sliced, ½ cup 5.8
Okra, frozen, boiled, drained, sliced, ½ cup 7.5
Olive, pickled:
    green, 10 small 4
    green, 10 giant 9
    green, pitted, 1 oz. 4
    green, stuffed with pimento, 1 oz. 1.7
    ripe, Greek, 10 medium 1.7
    ripe, Greek, pitted, 1 oz. 2.5
    ripe, Manzanilla or Mission, pitted, 1 oz. 1.8
    ripe, Sevillano or Ascolano, pitted, 1 oz. 1.6
Olive loaf, pork, 2 oz. 2.0
Onion, mature:
    raw, chopped, ¼ cup 3.5
    boiled, drained, chopped, ½ cup 10.7
    boiled, drained, chopped, 1 tbsp. 1.5
Onion, cocktail, 1 oz. 1.0
Onion, dried:
    flakes, 1 tbsp. 4.2
    minced, 1 tsp. 1.9
Onion, frozen (see also "Onion rings"):
    whole, boiled, drained, ½ cup 7.0
    chopped, boiled, drained, 1 tbsp. 1.0
Onion, green, raw, trimmed, with top:
    chopped, ½ cup 3.7
    chopped, 1 tbsp. 4

Onion, Welsh, 1 oz. 1.8
Onion dip, 2 tbsp. 2.5
Onion powder, 1 tsp. 1.7
Onion rings, frozen, breaded, heated, 10 rings 27.1
Onion salt, 1 tsp. 4
Orange, fresh:
    all varieties, sections, 1 cup 21.2
    California navel, 2⅞" fruit, 5 oz. 16.3
    California Valencia, 2⅝" fruit, 4.25 oz. 14.4
    Florida, 2¹¹⁄₁₆" fruit, 5 oz. 16.3
Orange, mandarin, see "Tangerine"
Orange drink, canned or bottled, 8 fl. oz. 32.0
Orange juice, 8 fl. oz.
    fresh 25.8
    chilled 25.1
    frozen, diluted 26.5
Orange peel, fresh, 1 tbsp. 1.5
Oregano, dried, 1 tsp. 5
Oriental 5-spice, 1 tsp. 1.9
Oyster, meat only:
    Eastern, wild, raw, 6 medium, 3 oz. 3.3
    Eastern, wild, baked or broiled, 4 oz. 5.4
    Eastern, wild, steamed or poached, 4 oz. 8.9
    Eastern, farmed, raw, 4 oz. 6.3
    Eastern, farmed, baked or broiled, 4 oz. 8.3
    Pacific, raw, 4 oz. 5.6
    Pacific, raw, steamed or poached, 1 medium........ 2.5
    Pacific, boiled or steamed, 4 oz. 11.2
Oyster, canned, Eastern, wild, with liquid, 4 oz. 4.4
Oyster plant, see "Salsify"
Oyster sauce, Asian, 1 tbsp. 2.0
Oyster stew, see "Soup, condensed"

P-Q

carbohydrates

Palm, hearts of, canned, 1.2-oz. piece 1.5
Pancake, frozen, plain, 4" cake 15.7
Pancake mix, prepared, 4" cake:
    plain 11.0
    plain, complete 14.0
    buckwheat 8.5
    whole wheat 13.0
Pancake syrup, 4 tbsp. or ¼ cup 53.0
Pancreas, without added ingredients 0
Panko flakes, ⅓ cup 15.0
Papaya, fresh:
    1 lb., 3½" x 5⅛" 29.8
    peeled, cubed, 1 cup 13.7

Papaya nectar, canned, 8 fl. oz. 36.3
Paprika, 1 tsp. 1.2
Parsley, fresh:
   10 sprigs 6
   chopped, ½ cup 1.9
Parsley, dried, 1 tbsp. 7
Parsnip, boiled, drained, sliced, ½ cup 15.2
Passion fruit, fresh, purple, trimmed, ½ cup 27.5
Passion fruit juice, fresh, purple, 8 fl. oz. 33.6
Pasta (see also "Macaroni"), cooked, 1 cup:
   corn 39.1
   spaghetti, plain 39.7
   spaghetti, protein fortified 44.3
   spaghetti, spinach 36.6
   spaghetti, whole wheat 37.2
Pasta, refrigerated, with egg, cooked, 4 oz. 28.3
Pasta sauce, tomato, ½ cup:
   marinara 12.7
   with mushrooms 10.3
   with onions 12.1
   with onion, green pepper, and celery 10.7
Pastrami, beef, 2 oz. 5
Pastry shell, see "Puff pastry"
Pâté, canned:
   chicken liver, 1 tbsp. 9
   goose liver, smoked, 1 tbsp. 6
Peach, fresh:
   2½" peach, 4 per lb. 9.7
   sliced, 1 cup 18.9
Peach, canned, halves or slices, ½ cup:
   in juice, with liquid 14.5
   in light syrup, with liquid 18.3
   in heavy syrup, with liquid 26.1
Peach, dried, sulfured, 5 halves, 2.3 oz. 39.8
Peach, frozen, sliced, sweetened, ½ cup 30.0
Peach nectar, canned, 8 fl. oz. 34.7
Peanut, shelled:
   raw, 1 oz. 4.5
   dry-roasted, ½ cup 15.7
   honey-roasted, 1 oz. 8.0
   oil-roasted, ½ cup 13.6
Peanut butter, 2 tbsp.:
   chunky style 6.9
   smooth or creamy style 6.6
Pear, fresh, with peel:
   1 large, 2 per lb. 31.6
   Bartlett, 1 medium, 2½ per lb. 25.1
   sliced, ½ cup 12.5
Pear, Asian, 1 medium, 2¼" x 2½" diam. 13.0

Pear, canned, halves or slices, ½ cup:

in juice, with liquid 16.0

in light syrup, with liquid 19.0

in heavy syrup, with liquid 25.5

Pear, dried, sulfured, halves, ½ cup 62.7

Pear nectar, canned, 8 fl. oz. 39.4

Peas, edible-podded, fresh:

raw, ½ cup 5.4

boiled, drained, ½ cup 5.6

Peas, edible-podded, frozen, boiled, drained,

½ cup 7.2

Peas, green, fresh:

raw, shelled, ½ cup 10.4

boiled, drained, ½ cup 12.5

Peas, green, canned, drained, ½ cup 10.7

Peas, green, frozen, boiled, drained, ½ cup 11.4

Peas, sugar snap or snow, see "Peas, edible-podded"

Peas, split, see "Split peas"

Peas and carrots, ½ cup:

canned, with liquid 11.0

frozen, boiled, drained 8.1

Peas and onions, ½ cup:

canned, with liquid 5.1

frozen, boiled, drained, ½ cup 7.8

Pecan, shelled:

1 oz. 5.2

halves, 1 cup 19.7

dry-roasted, 1 cup 14.9

oil-roasted, 1 cup 14.3

Pepeao, raw, sliced, 1 cup 6.7

Pepeao, dried, 1 cup 19.5

Pepper, seasoning:

black or white, ground, 1 tsp. 1.7

chili, 1 tsp. 1.2

red or cayenne, 1 tsp. 1.0

Pepper, ancho, dried, .6-oz. pepper 8.7

Pepper, banana, fresh, 1.2-oz. piece 1.8

Pepper, chili, fresh, green and red:

1 medium, 1.6 oz. 4.3

chopped, ½ cup 7.1

Pepper, chili, canned, 1 large, 2.6 oz. 3.7

Pepper, chili, dried, sun-dried, hot, 2 pieces 8

Pepper, green or red, sweet, see "Pepper, sweet"

Pepper, jalapeño, fresh, .5-oz. piece 8

Pepper, jalapeño, canned, sliced, with liquid,

¼ cup 1.6

Pepper, Serrano, fresh, .2-oz. piece 4

Pepper, sweet, fresh:

raw, 1 medium, 3¾" x 3", or ½ cup chopped 4.8

raw, sliced, 1 cup 5.9
boiled, drained, chopped, 1 tbsp. 8
boiled, drained, strips, ½ cup 4.6
yellow, raw, 1 large, 5" x 3" 11.8
yellow, raw, 10 strips, 1.8 oz. 3.3
Pepper, sweet, canned, red, drained, ½ cup 2.7
Pepper, sweet, freeze-dried, red or green,
¼ cup 1.1
Pepper, sweet, frozen, chopped, 1 oz. 1.2
Pepperoni, pork and beef, 1 oz. 8
Perch, without added ingredients 0
Persimmon, fresh:
Japanese, 1 medium 31.2
native, 1 medium, 1.1 oz. 8.4
Pesto sauce, basil, in jars, ¼ cup 3.5
Pheasant, without added ingredients 0
Pickle, cucumber:
bread and butter, 1 oz. 6.0
dill, 3¾" long, 2.3 oz. 2.7
sour, 3¾" long, 1.2 oz. 8
sweet, 3" long, 1.2 oz. 11.1
Pickle and pimento loaf, 2 oz. 3.5
Pickle relish, cucumber, 1 tbsp.:
hamburger 5.2
hot dog 3.5
sweet 5.3
Pickling spice, 1 tsp. 1.2
Pie, commercial:
apple, ⅛ of 9" pie 42.5
blueberry, ⅛ of 9" pie 43.7
cherry, ⅛ of 9" pie 49.8
chocolate cream, ⅙ of 8" pie 37.9
coconut custard, ⅙ of 8" pie 31.5
lemon meringue, ⅙ of 8" pie 53.3
peach, ⅙ of 8" pie 38.5
pecan, ⅙ of 8" pie 64.7
pumpkin, ⅙ of 8" pie 29.8
Pie, snack, fruit, fried, 4-oz. piece 48.3
Pie crust, frozen, 9" shell 62.7
Pie crust mix, prepared, 9" shell 80.7
Pie filling, canned, fruit, ⅓ cup 24.0
Pig's feet, pickled, cured, 1 oz. .... <.1
Pigeon peas, fresh, boiled, drained, ½ cup 15.0
Pigeon peas, dried, boiled, ½ cup 19.5
Pignolia nuts, see "Pine nuts"
Pike, without added ingredients 0
Pili nuts, shelled, dried, ½ cup 2.4
Pine nuts, dried:
pignolia, 1 oz. 4.0

pinyon, 1 oz. 5.5
pinyon, 10 kernels 2
Pineapple, fresh:
    3½" slice, 3 oz. 10.4
    diced, ½ cup 9.6
Pineapple, canned, ½ cup:
    in juice, chunks or tidbits 19.6
    in light syrup, crushed or chunks 17.0
    in heavy syrup, chunks, tidbits, or crushed 25.8
Pineapple, frozen, chunks, sweetened, ½ cup 27.1
Pineapple juice, canned or bottled, 8 fl. oz. 34.5
Pink beans, dried, boiled, ½ cup 23.5
Pinto beans, boiled, ½ cup 21.8
Pinto beans, canned, with liquid, ½ cup 17.5
Pistachio nut:
    dried, in shell, 4 oz. 14.1
    dried, shelled, 1 oz. 7.1
    dry-roasted, in shell, 4 oz. 16.2
    dry-roasted, shelled, 1 oz. 7.8
Pitanga, 1 medium, .3 oz. 5
Pizza, cheese, frozen, ¼ of 16-oz. pie 32.8
Pizza sauce, canned, ¼ cup 6.0
Plantain, fresh:
    raw, 1 medium, 6.3 oz. 57.1
    cooked, sliced, ½ cup 24.0
Plum, fresh:
    Japanese or hybrid, 2⅛" fruit 8.6
    sliced, ½ cup 10.7
Plum, canned, purple, ½ cup:
    in juice 19.1
    in light syrup 20.5
    in heavy syrup 30.0
Plum, dried (prune):
    10 pieces 52.7
    with pits, ½ cup 50.5
    stewed, with pits, unsweetened, ½ cup 29.8
Plum, dried, canned, in heavy syrup:
    ½ cup 32.5
    5 pieces and 2 tbsp. liquid 23.9
Poi, ½ cup 32.7
Pokeberry shoots, raw, ½ cup 3.0
Polenta (see also "Cornmeal"), prepared, 3.5 oz. 15.0
Pollock, without added ingredients 0
Pomegranate, with peel, 9.7-oz. fruit 26.4
Pomegranate juice, bottled, 8 fl. oz. 36.5
Pompano, Florida, without added ingredients 0
Popcorn, popped:
    air-popped, 3 cups 18.0
    oil-popped, 3 cups 18.5

caramel coated, with peanuts, 2 oz. 45.7
Popcorn cakes, 2 cakes, .75 oz. 16.0
Poppy seeds, 1 tsp. 7
Pork, fresh, meat only, without added ingredients 0
Pork, cured (see also "Ham"):
    arm (picnic), roasted, 4 oz. 0
    blade roll, lean with fat, roasted, 4 oz. 4
Pork backfat or belly, 2 oz. 0
Pork lunch meat, oven-roasted, 2 oz. 1.0
Pork rind snack, 1 oz. 5
Potato:
    raw, unpeeled, 1 large, 6.5 oz. 33.1
    baked, in skin, 4¾" x 2" 51.0
    baked, without skin, ½ cup 13.2
    baked, skin only, 1 oz. 13.1
    boiled in skin, peeled, 2½" potato, 4.8 oz. 27.4
    boiled in skin, peeled, ½ cup 15.7
    boiled without skin, 2½" potato 27.0
    boiled without skin, ½ cup 15.6
    mashed, with whole milk, ½ cup 18.4
    mashed, with milk and butter or margarine,
    ½ cup 17.5
Potato, canned:
    drained, 1 cup 24.5
    whole, 1.2-oz. potato 4.8
Potato, frozen:
    French fried, oven-heated, 10 strips, 1.75 oz. 17.0
    fried, cottage cut, oven-heated, 4 oz. 38.6
    hash brown, prepared in oil, ½ cup 21.9
    puffs, oven-heated, ½ cup 18.9
Potato, sweet, see "Sweet potato"
Potato chips or sticks, 1 oz. 15.0
Poultry seasoning, 1 tsp. 1.0
Pout, ocean, without added ingredients 0
Pretzels, 1 oz. 22.0
Prickly pear, 4.8-oz. fruit, 3.6 oz. trimmed 9.9
Prosciutto, 2 oz. 0
Prune, see "Plum, dried"
Prune juice, canned, 8 fl. oz. 44.7
Pudding (see also "Custard"), ready-to-eat, 4 oz.:
    banana 24.0
    chocolate 26.0
    lemon 28.5
    rice 25.0
    tapioca 22.0
    vanilla 24.8
Pudding mix, prepared with milk, ½ cup:
    banana, instant 29.0
    banana, regular 25.3

chocolate, instant 27.8
chocolate, regular 25.5
coconut cream, instant 28.0
coconut cream, regular 24.7
lemon, instant 29.5
rice 30.0
tapioca 27.6
vanilla, instant 27.9
vanilla, regular 26.0
Puff pastry, frozen, 1.4-oz. shell 18.3
Pummelo, sections, 1 cup 18.3
Pumpkin, fresh, boiled, drained, mashed, ½ cup 6.0
Pumpkin, canned, with or without squash, ½ cup 9.9
Pumpkin flower, boiled, drained, ½ cup 2.2
Pumpkin pie spice, 1 tsp. 1.2
Pumpkin seeds:
dried, shelled, 1 oz. or 142 kernels 5.1
roasted, in shell, 1 oz. or 85 seeds 15.3
roasted, shelled, 1 oz. 3.8
Purslane, boiled, drained, ½ cup 2.1
Quail, meat only, without added ingredients 0
Quince, 1 medium, 5.3 oz. 14.1
Quinoa, dry, ¼ cup 29.3

R
carbohydrates

Rabbit, meat only, without added ingredients 0
Radicchio, fresh:
1 medium leaf, .3 oz. 4
shredded, 1 cup 1.8
Radish, raw, 10 medium, ¾"–1" diam. 1.6
Radish, Oriental:
raw, 7" piece, 11.9 oz. 12.8
raw, sliced, ½ cup 1.8
boiled, drained, sliced, ½ cup 2.5
Radish, white-icicle, 1 medium, .6 oz. 5
Raisins, seedless, not packed, ¼ cup 28.7
Rapini, see "Broccoli rabe"
Raspberry, fresh, ½ cup 7.1
Raspberry, frozen, sweetened, ½ cup 32.7
Red beans (see also "Kidney beans"), canned,
½ cup 19.0
Red snapper or redfish, without added ingredients 0
Refried beans, canned, ½ cup 23.3
Rhubarb, fresh, 1 medium stalk 2.3
Rice (see also "Wild rice"), cooked, ½ cup:
brown, long grain 22.5
white, long grain 22.3

white, long grain, parboiled 21.7
white, long grain, precooked or instant 17.4
Rice cake (see also "Popcorn cakes"), .7-oz. piece   15.0
Rice flour:
brown, ¼ cup 30.2
white, ¼ cup 31.7
Rockfish, without added ingredients 0
Roe (see also "Caviar"), mixed species:
raw, 1 oz. or 2 tbsp. 4
baked or broiled, 2 oz. 1.0
Roll (see also "Biscuit"), 1 roll:
brown and serve or plain, 2 oz. 28.6
egg, 2 oz. 29.5
French, 2 oz. 28.5
hamburger or hot dog, 2 oz. 28.5
hot dog, mixed grain, 2 oz. 25.3
kaiser or hard, 3½" roll, 2 oz. 29.9
oat bran, 2 oz. 22.8
rye, 2 oz. 30.1
wheat, 2 oz. 26.1
wheat, whole, 2 oz. 29.0
Roselle, 1 oz. or ½ cup 3.2
Rosemary, fresh, .5 oz. 3.0
Rosemary, dried, 1 tsp. 8
Roughy, orange, without added ingredients 0
Rutabaga, fresh:
boiled, drained, cubed, ½ cup 7.4
boiled, drained, mashed, ½ cup 10.5
Rye flour, medium, ¼ cup 20.0

S

Sablefish, without added ingredients 0
Safflower kernels, dried, 1 oz. 9.7
Safflower meal, partially defatted, 1 oz. 13.8
Saffron, 1 tsp. 5
Sage, ground, 1 tsp. 4
Salad dressing, 2 tbsp.:
blue cheese 2.2
Caesar 2.0
French 5.4
French, low-calorie 7.0
Italian 3.0
mayonnaise type 7.0
ranch 2.0
Russian 9.0
Thousand Island 4.8
Salami, 2 oz.:

beef, cooked 1.4
beef and pork, cooked 1.2
pork, dry or hard 1.0
pork and beef, dry or hard 1.5
Salmon, fresh or canned, without added
    ingredients 0
Salmon, smoked, 2 oz. 1
Salsa, 2 tbsp. 2.0
Salsify, boiled, drained, sliced, ½ cup 10.5
Salt, regular or seasoned, 1 tbsp. 0
Salt pork, raw 0
Sandwich spread, 1 tbsp.:
    beef and pork 1.8
    meatless, mayonnaise type 3.0
Sapodilla, pulp, ½ cup 24.1
Sapote, 11.2-oz. fruit, 7.9 oz. trimmed 76.0
Sardine, fresh 0
Sardine, canned:
    in oil, 4 oz. 0
    in tomato or mustard sauce, 2 oz. or ¼ cup 1.0
Sauerkraut, canned, with liquid, ¼ cup 5.0
Sausage (see also specific listings), pork:
    4" link cooked, yield from 1-oz. raw 1
    1-oz. patty cooked, yield from 2 oz. raw 3
    Italian, cooked, 2 oz. 8
    smoked, 2 oz. 1.2
"Sausage," vegetarian:
    .9-oz. link 2.5
    1.3-oz. patty 3.7
Sausage seasoning, 1 tsp. 2.7
Sausage stick, smoked, 1 oz. 1.5
Savory, ground, 1 tsp. 1.0
Scallion, see "Onion, green"
Scallop, meat only:
    raw, 2 large or 5 small, 1.1 oz. 7
    steamed, 4 oz. 0
Scallop squash, ½ cup:
    boiled, drained, sliced 3.0
    boiled, drained, mashed 4.0
Scrapple, 2 oz. 6.0
Scrod or scup, without added ingredients 0
Sea bass or sea trout, without added ingredients 0
Seafood sauce, cocktail, ¼ cup 16.0
Semolina, whole-grain, ¼ cup 30.4
Sesame meal, partially defatted, 1 oz. 7.4
Sesame paste, from whole seeds, 1 tbsp. 4.1
Sesame seeds:
    dried, 1 tbsp. 2.1
    roasted, toasted, 1 oz 7.3

Shad, without added ingredients 0
Shallot, fresh, chopped, 1 tbsp. 1.7
Shallot, freeze-dried, 1 tbsp. 7
Shark or sheepshead, without added ingredients 0
Shellie beans, canned with liquid, ½ cup 7.6
Sherbet, orange, ½ cup 29.2
Sherbet bar, orange, 2.75-fl.oz. bar 20.1
Shortening, 1 cup 0
Shrimp, fresh, meat only:
    raw, 4 large, 1 oz. 3
    boiled or steamed, 4 oz. 0
Shrimp, canned, drained:, 1 cup 1.3
"Shrimp," imitation, from surimi, 4 oz. 10.4
Smelt, rainbow, without added ingredients 0
Snail, fresh, raw, 1 oz. .... <.1
Snail, sea, see "Whelk"
Snapper, without added ingredients 0
Snow peas, see "Peas, edible-podded"
Soft drinks, carbonated, 12 fl. oz.:
    club soda or seltzer 0
    cola 42.0
    ginger ale 38.0
    orange 52.0
    root beer 43.0
    tonic 36.0
Sole, without added ingredients 0
Sorbet, raspberry, ½ cup 30.0
Sorghum syrup, 1 tbsp. 15.7
Sorrel, see "Dock"
Soup, ready-to-serve, 1 cup:
    bean, black 28.0
    bean with ham, chunky 27.1
    beef 19.6
    beef or chicken broth 1
    chicken, chunky 17.3
    chicken noodle 15.0
    chicken rice, chunky 13.0
    chicken vegetable, chunky 19.0
    clam chowder, Manhattan or New England 18.9
    lentil with ham 20.2
    minestrone, chunky 20.7
    vegetable, chunky 19.0
Soup, condensed, diluted with water, 1 cup:
    bean with bacon 22.8
    beef broth or bouillon 1.0
    broccoli cheese 12.0
    cheese 10.5
    chicken broth 9
    chicken and dumplings 6.0

chicken gumbo 8.4
chicken noodle 9.4
chicken rice 7.2
chicken vegetable 8.6
chili beef 21.5
clam chowder, Manhattan 12.2
minestrone 11.2
mushroom, with beef stock 9.3
onion 8.2
oyster stew, diluted with whole milk 9.8
pea, green 26.5
pea, split, with ham 28.0
tomato 16.6
tomato beef with noodles 21.2
tomato rice 21.9
turkey noodle or vegetable 8.6
vegetable beef 10.2
vegetarian vegetable 13.0
Soup mix, prepared with water, 1 cup:
beef broth or bouillon 1.9
beef noodle 6.0
chicken broth or bouillon 1.4
chicken noodle 7.4
leek 11.4
minestrone 11.9
mushroom 11.1
onion 5.1
pea, green or split 22.7
tomato or cream of tomato 19.4
vegetable beef 8.0
Sour cream, see "Cream, sour"
Soursop, ½ cup 18.9
Soy milk:
8 fl. oz. 14.2
calcium fortified, 8 fl. oz. 8.4
Soy nuts, roasted, toasted, ½ cup 16.5
Soy protein, concentrate, 1 oz. 8.8
Soy sauce, 1 tbsp.:
from soy (tamari) 1.0
from soy and wheat (shoyu) 1.5
low sodium 2.0
Soybeans, fresh:
raw, shelled, ½ cup 14.1
boiled, drained, ½ cup 10.0
Soybeans, dried, boiled, ½ cup 8.5
Soybeans, roasted, ½ cup 28.9
Soybean curd or cake, see "Tofu"
Soybean flour, stirred, ¼ cup:
defatted 9.6

low fat 8.4
Soybean sprouts, steamed, ½ cup 3.1
Spaghetti, see "Pasta"
Spaghetti sauce, see "Pasta sauce"
Spaghetti squash, baked or boiled, drained, ½ cup .. 5.0
Spelt, grain, ¼ cup 32.0
Spinach, fresh:
   raw, chopped, ½ cup 1.0
   cooked, boiled, drained, ½ cup boiled 3.4
Spinach, canned, drained, ½ cup 3.6
Spinach, frozen, chopped or leaf, drained, ½ cup 5.1
Spinach, malabar, cooked, 1 cup 1.2
Spinach, New Zealand, boiled, drained, ½ cup 2.0
Spiny lobster, meat only:
   boiled or steamed, 2 lbs. in shell 5.1
   boiled or steamed, 4 oz. 3.5
Spleen, braised, without added ingredients 0
Split peas, boiled, ½ cup 20.7
Spot, without added ingredients 0
Sprouts, see "Bean sprouts" and specific listings
Squab, meat only, without added ingredients 0
Squid, fresh, meat only, raw, 4 oz. 3.5
Star fruit, see "Carambola"
Strawberry, fresh, trimmed, ½ cup 5.2
Strawberry, canned, in heavy syrup, ½ cup 29.9
Strawberry, frozen, unsweetened, ½ cup 10.1
Strawberry syrup, 2 tbsp. 26.0
String beans, see "Green beans"
Stuffing mix, bread, dry, 1 oz. 21.6
Sturgeon, without added ingredients 0
Succotash, canned, ½ cup:
   kernels 17.9
   cream-style 23.4
Succotash, frozen, boiled, drained, ½ cup 17.0
Sucker, white, without added ingredients 0
Sugar, beet or cane:
   granulated, 1 tbsp. 12.0
   granulated, 1 tsp. 4.0
   powdered/confectioner's, unsifted, 1 tbsp. 8.0
Sugar, maple, 1 oz. 25.5
Sugar, substitute, 1 pkt. .... <1.0
Sugar apple, 1 medium, 9.9 oz. 36.6
Sugar snap peas, see "Peas, edible-podded"
Summer sausage, 2 oz. 1.0
Sunfish, pumpkinseed, without added ingredients 0
Sunflower butter, 1 tbsp. 4.4
Sunflower seed flour, partially defatted, 1 cup 28.7
Surimi, pollock, 4 oz. 7.8
Swamp cabbage, boiled, drained, chopped, ½ cup 1.8

Sweet peas, see "Peas, green"
Sweet potato:
    baked in skin, 5" x 2" potato 27.7
    baked in skin, mashed, ½ cup 24.3
    boiled, without skin, 4 oz. 20.1
    boiled, without skin, mashed, ½ cup 31.7
Sweet potato, canned, ½ cup:
    cut, vacuum packed 21.1
    in syrup, with liquid 23.9
    in syrup, drained 24.9
Sweet and sour sauce, Chinese style, 1 tbsp. 7.0
Sweetbreads, without added ingredients 0
Swiss chard, fresh:
    raw, chopped, ½ cup 7
    boiled, drained, chopped, ½ cup 3.6
Swordfish, without added ingredients 0

T

carbohydrates

Taco sauce, 1 tbsp. 1.5
Taco shell, 3 average 19.0
Tahini, sesame, from roasted kernels, 1 tbsp. 3.2
Tamarind:
    1 fruit, 3" x 1" 1.3
    pulp, ½ cup 37.5
Tangerine, fresh:
    1 large 2½" diam., 3.5 oz. 11.0
    sections, 1 cup 21.8
Tangerine, canned (mandarin orange):
    in juice, with liquid, ½ cup 11.9
    in light syrup, with liquid, ½ cup 20.4
Tangerine juice, 8 fl. oz.:
    fresh 25.0
    canned, sweetened 29.9
Tapioca, dry, pearl, 1 tbsp. 10.0
Tapioca pudding, see "Pudding"
Taro, cooked, sliced, ½ cup 22.8
Taro, Tahitian, cooked, sliced, ½ cup 4.7
Taro chips, 1 oz. 19.3
Taro leaf, steamed, ½ cup 2.9
Taro shoots, cooked, sliced, ½ cup 2.2
Tarragon, ground, 1 tsp. 8
Tartar sauce, 2 tbsp. 2.0
Tea, plain, regular or herbal, bag or 1 tsp. 0
Tempeh, 1 oz. 2.7
Teriyaki sauce, 1 tbsp. 3.0
Thyme, ground, 1 tsp. 9
Thymus, beef or veal, without added ingredients 0

Tilapia, without added ingredients 0
Tilefish, without added ingredients 0
Tofu (see also "Tempeh"):
    fresh, firm, ½ cup 5.4
    fresh, soft, ½ cup 2.3
    okara, ½ cup 7.7
    salted and fermented (fuyu), 1 oz. 1.5
Tomatillo, fresh:
    1 medium, 1⅜" diam. 2.0
    chopped, ½ cup 3.8
Tomato, fresh, ripe:
    raw, 1 medium, 2⅗" diam., 4.75 oz. 5.7
    raw, chopped, 1 cup 8.4
    boiled, 1 cup 14.0
    orange, 3.9-oz. tomato 3.5
    yellow, 7.8-oz. tomato 6.3
Tomato, canned, ½ cup:
    whole, peeled 5.2
    wedges, in tomato juice or stewed 8.3
    diced 6.0
    with green chilies 4.3
Tomato, dried:
    1 piece, 32 pieces per cup 1.1
    ½ cup 15.3
Tomato, green, raw, 1 large, 6.4 oz. 9.3
Tomato juice, 8 fl. oz. 10.0
Tomato paste, 2 tbsp. 6.0
Tomato puree, ¼ cup 6.0
Tomato sauce (see also "Pasta sauce"), canned:
    regular or Spanish style, ½ cup 8.8
    with onions, ½ cup 12.1
    with tomato tidbits, ½ cup 8.7
Tomato-beef drink, 8 fl. oz. 11.0
Tongue, beef, braised, 4 oz. 4
Tortilla chips, see "Corn chips/crisps"
Trail mix, 1 oz.:
    regular, plain or with chocolate chips 12.7
    tropical mix 18.6
Trout, without added ingredients 0
Tuna, fresh or canned, without added ingredients 0
Turbot, without added ingredients 0
Turkey, meat only, without added ingredients 0
Turkey giblets, simmered, diced, 1 cup 3.0
Turkey gravy, canned, ¼ cup 3.5
Turkey lunch meat, breast, oven-roasted, 2 oz. 1.0
Turkey salami, cooked, 1 oz. 2
Turmeric, ground, 1 tsp. 1.4
Turnip:
    boiled, drained, cubed, ½ cup 3.8

boiled, drained, mashed, ½ cup 5.6
Turnip, frozen, boiled, drained, ½ cup 3.4
Turnip greens, fresh:
    raw, chopped, ½ cup 1.6
    boiled, chopped, ½ cup 3.1
Turnip greens, canned, with liquid, ½ cup 2.8
Turnip greens, frozen, boiled, drained, 1 cup 4.7

V–W

Vanilla extract, imitation:
    with alcohol, 1 tbsp. 3
    without alcohol, 1 tbsp. 1.8
Veal, meat only, without added ingredients 0
Vegetable juice, 8 fl. oz. 10.0
Vegetables, see specific listings
Vegetables, mixed, canned, with liquid, ½ cup 8.7
Vegetables, mixed, frozen, boiled, drained,
    ½ cup 11.9
Venison, meat only, without added ingredients 0
Vienna sausage, beef and pork, 2" link 3
Vinegar, 1 tbsp. 1.0
Waffle, frozen, 4"-square piece 13.5
Waffle mix, see "Pancake mix"
Walnut, dried, shelled:
    black, 1 oz. 3.4
    black, chopped, 1 cup 15.1
    English or Persian, 1 oz. 5.2
    English or Persian, halves, 1 cup 18.3
Wasabi powder, 1 tsp. 1.0
Water chestnut, fresh:
    4 medium, 1.3 oz. 8.6
    sliced, ½ cup 14.8
Water chestnut, canned:
    whole, 4 pieces, 1 oz. 3.5
    sliced, with liquid, ½ cup 8.7
Watercress, 10 sprigs or ½ cup chopped 3
Watermelon, fresh:
    1 slice, 1" thick x 10" diam. 34.6
    diced, ½ cup 5.7
Watermelon seeds, dried, 1 oz. 4.4
Wax beans, see "Green beans"
Wax gourd, boiled, drained, cubed, 1 cup 5.3
Wheat, whole grain, ¼ cup 33.0
Wheat, parboiled, see "Bulgur"
Wheat, sprouted, 1 cup 45.9
Wheat berries, see "Wheat kernels"
Wheat bran, coarse or crude, ¼ cup 10.0

Wheat flour, ¼ cup:
    all purpose, white 23.9
    cake, white 21.3
    self-rising, white 23.2
    tortilla mix 18.6
    whole grain 21.8
Wheat germ:
    crude, 2 tbsp. 14.0
    toasted, 3 tbsp. 12.0
Wheat kernels, ¼ cup 34.5
Whelk, meat only, boiled or steamed, 4 oz. 17.6
Whey, fluid, acid or sweet, 1 cup 12.6
White beans, mature, boiled, ½ cup 22.6
White beans, canned, with liquid, ½ cup 28.7
Whitefish, fresh or smoked, without added
    ingredients 0
Whiting, without added ingredients 0
Wiener, see "Frankfurter"
Wild rice, cooked, 1 cup 35.0
Wine, 3.5 fl. oz., except as noted:
    dessert/aperitif (port, sherry, vermouth, etc.) 12.2
    dry or table, red 1.8
    dry or table, rosé 1.4
    dry or table, white 8
    sake 5
Winged beans, fresh, raw or boiled, drained,
    ½ cup 1.0
Winged beans, mature, boiled, ½ cup 12.8
Winged bean tuber, trimmed, 1 oz. 8.0
Wolf fish, without added ingredients 0
Wonton wrapper, 3.5"-square piece 4.6
Worcestershire sauce, 1 tsp. 1.0

Y–Z   carbohydrates

Yachtwurst, with pistachios, cooked, 2 oz. 8
Yam, baked or boiled, cubed, ½ cup 18.8
Yam, canned or frozen, see "Sweet potato"
Yam, mountain, steamed, cubed, ½ cup 14.4
Yam beans, tuber:
    raw, sliced, ½ cup 5.3
    boiled, drained, 4 oz. 10.0
Yard-long beans:
    fresh, boiled, drained, sliced, ½ cup 4.8
    mature, boiled, ½ cup 18.1
Yeast, baker's, ¼ oz. 2.7
Yellow beans, dried, boiled, ½ cup 22.2
Yellowtail, without added ingredients 0

Yogurt, 8 oz.:

    plain, whole milk 10.6

    plain, low fat 16.0

    plain, nonfat or skim 17.4

    with fruit, low fat 43.0

Yogurt, frozen, chocolate, ½ cup 18.8

Yogurt, tofu, ½ cup 20.9

Yuca, boiled, drained, 4 oz. 38.6

Zucchini, fresh, with skin:

    raw, sliced, ½ cup 1.6

    raw, baby, 1 large, 3⅛" 5

    boiled, drained, sliced, ½ cup 3.5

Zucchini, canned, with tomato juice, ½ cup 7.8

Zucchini, frozen, with skin, boiled, drained, 1 cup .. 7.9